EVERYTHING YOU NEED TO KNOW ABOUT

BIRD 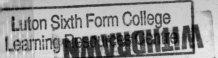 FLU

& WHAT YOU CAN DO TO PREPARE FOR IT

EVERYTHING YOU NEED TO KNOW ABOUT

BIRD✚FLU

& WHAT YOU CAN DO TO PREPARE FOR IT

JO REVILL

RODALE®

This edition first published in the UK in 2005 by
Rodale International Ltd
7–10 Chandos Street
London W1G 9AD
www.rodalebooks.co.uk

The moral right of Jo Revill to be identified as the author or this work has been asserted in
accordance with the Copyright, Designs and Patents Act of 1988.

Book design by Paul Ashby

Illustrations on p.30 and p.62 by Michael Agar; illustrations on p. 96 and pp.182–187 by
Paul Ashby

Author photograph by Susanne Blankemeyer

Printed and bound in the UK by CPI Bath using acid-free paper
from sustainable sources.

3 5 7 9 8 6 4 2

A CIP record for this book is available from the British Library

ISBN-13 978-1-4050-9573-0
ISBN-10 1-4050-9573-3

This paperback edition distributed to the book trade by Pan Macmillan Ltd

Notice
This book is intended as a reference volume only, not a medical manual. The information
given here is designed to help you make informed decisions about your health. It is not
intended as a substitute for any treatment that may have been prescribed by your doctor. If
you suspect that you have a medical problem, we urge you to seek competent medical help.

Mention of specific companies, organizations or authorities in this book does not imply
endorsement by the publisher, nor does mention of specific companies, organizations or
authorities in the book imply that they endorse the book.

Websites and telephone numbers given in this book were accurate at the time the book
went to press.

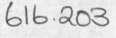

RODALE
LIVE YOUR WHOLE LIFE™

10061807

To my father, who showed us all such wisdom and love

CONTENTS

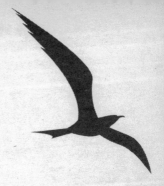

ACKNOWLEDGEMENTS

'Aren't you sick of bird flu?' friends would ask when we met for coffee, as I groaned about the labour pains of book-writing. The strange thing is that I'm still as fascinated by the subject as I was when I began, largely thanks to all the people who've generously given their time and shared their wisdom with me.

So many scientists and doctors have helped with this book that it's hard to know where to begin, but above all, I must thank Professor John Oxford and Professor Peter Openshaw for their guidance in steering me through the twilight world of virology. Officials at the Department of Health and the Health Protection Agency have also been very helpful, far more so than they needed to be.

I'm lucky to have had Rob Shreeve as my agent. In the past few months, he has steered me on a whirlwind course through the complexities of publishing with humour and very constructive advice. Liz Coghill, my editor at Rodale, has shown great patience with me, coupled with an enormous interest in the subject itself, and I would like to thank everyone at Rodale for their help.

I also owe a lot to my copy-editor Gill Paul and to Michael Agar, who drew the diagrams. My friend Susanne Blankemeyer provided the lunches, the digital camera and her usual sound advice.

Colleagues at the *Observer*, while not quite sharing my obsession, have nevertheless been extremely supportive. I'd like to thank my editor Roger Alton and deputy editor Paul Webster for allowing me time off to write the book. Robin McKie, Anushka Asthana and Amelia Hill were unfailingly generous and helpful colleagues.

My mother Diane Revill read the early chapters and has always been supportive from the very start. But, above all, it is to my husband, Michael McCarthy, that I owe more than I can say. His thoughtfulness, along with all those late-night conversations about chicken farms, made it possible for me to write the book. Flora and Seb, I promise never to mention flu masks again.

FOREWORD

by Professor Peter Openshaw

For each of the past four winters, news headlines have been grabbed by reports of new viral threats. The current anxiety over avian influenza is not due to scaremongering by scientists or others with a vested interest in creating hype. With a mixture of alarm and fascination we are, for the first time, witnessing the emergence of the largest outbreak of influenza ever seen in birds, both wild and domestic.

The geographic spread of the H5N1 subtype is unprecedented, as is its range of hosts. It has already infected large cats and some humans, causing a 50 per cent death rate. Adding to our anxiety comes the discovery that the Spanish flu that killed so many people just after World War I was due to a cross-species jump of a similar bird virus that, suddenly and without warning, mutated and spread between people and around the globe.

And since 1918, opportunities for pandemic viruses seem to have improved. The human population has been growing at an alarming rate, with an increasing concentration of people in dense urban environments. Flu viruses spread easily between people living in air-conditioned spaces, travelling in crowded buses, visiting cinemas and theatres and being confined in ever-larger aeroplanes.

If viruses were able to think or develop a strategy, there could be none better than to spread through air, food or water; indeed, most viruses seem to have evolved to take advantage of our need to breathe, eat and drink. Of course, viruses do not plan, but use their rapid evolutionary ability to exploit changes in human behaviour. As we change the way we live, so viruses adapt and evolve with us.

There are two types of virus and they adopt different strategies: DNA viruses are relatively stable, lumbering beasts, while the RNA viruses mutate fast, generating many new variants each time they hijack a cell. Each infected cell makes hundreds or thousands of viral offspring, each subtly different and competing against its siblings for survival. That is why scientists become alarmed when they see the levels of an RNA virus like H5N1 rising like floodwater in both domestic poultry and migratory birds.

There are puzzling differences between the way that ordinary human flu and bird flu affect us. With ordinary flu, those already weakened by old age, disease and debility are the first to die. Being unable to mount a sufficiently vigorous immune response seems to make people vulnerable to complications like pneumonia. But people who die from bird flu tend to be young or in the prime of life, mostly aged between ten and 22 years; they die from a combination of respiratory failure, circulatory collapse and renal failure in the second to fourth week of disease, sometimes despite full treatment with anti-viral drugs. This seems to result from a catastrophic over-reaction by a vigorous immune system – quite different to the situation with ordinary flu. Part of the problem is that we still don't really understand why young, healthy people suffer from multiple organ failure after bird flu infection, or how to treat it.

Our concerns about bird flu are fed by an unprecedented deluge of facts. There has been an extraordinary acceleration in what we know about viruses, the speed with which they can be discovered and the ease with which their genetic code can be deciphered. Scientific advances in interpreting this information have also been remarkable, from the generation of computer models of the molecular engagement of viral proteins with host cells, through to predictive maps of the global spread of disease.

In addition, the willingness of scientists and politicians to pass information on to the general public has grown. It is no longer possible or acceptable to filter what an increasingly sophisticated public should be told. Indeed, politicians and scientists are well aware that concealing the facts is almost always unwise and doomed to failure. If the facts are not passed on, information and rumour will soon spread via the media and the Internet. It is much better to present the facts honestly, quickly and accurately.

This book is an accessible guide to avian flu, summarizing what the public needs to know and how they can prepare. Inevitably, there are uncertainties. Until the virus has mutated and is starting to spread between humans, we have no idea how bad an epidemic will be. Sometimes, mutations that allow spread in a new species reduce disease severity, but until the mutation happens we just don't know.

In the run-up to a flu epidemic, it is vital that we have a well-informed, educated public that can make sound judgements, respond appropriately and evaluate the uncertainties intelligently. This timely book should be invaluable in preparing for an outbreak – perhaps this winter, perhaps the next, but surely at some time in the not too distant future.

Peter Openshaw
MB BS BSc PhD FRCP FMedSci
Professor of Experimental Medicine
Head, Section of Respiratory Infections
National Heart and Lung Division
Imperial College, London

Friday, 11 November 2005

NOTE ON THE AUTHOR:
Peter Openshaw is a Consultant in Respiratory Medicine at St Mary's Hospital, Paddington. He has been working on respiratory viruses since 1985, and established the Department of Respiratory Medicine in 1988. He is supported by the Wellcome Trust and leads a team of 40 scientists working on respiratory viruses, as well as teaching at Imperial College, London.

INTRODUCTION

Bird flu. Two little words – but what an impact they have made upon the world. In the last two years, we have seen country after country struggling in vain to eradicate a virus that has leapt across national boundaries to infect countless millions of chickens and geese. At the moment it is still a disease of birds, but the great fear is that it will evolve into an infection that is contagious between human beings, which could cause a worldwide flu pandemic. We have already seen alarming TV bulletins showing the first victims, mostly healthy, young people, struggling to catch their breath as their lungs become clouded over with the infection.

Every 30 to 50 years, influenza sweeps across the planet, taking advantage of the fact that our immune system is not able to recognize new strains of the virus. If we are lucky, the next global outbreak will be mild. But if the current strain of bird flu forms the next pandemic, as seems likely, the implications will be very serious.

There's a chance that the virus which is causing so much concern – a flu subtype known as H5N1 – may never become 'humanized' (in other words, able to pass from human to human), but that possibility is receding fast, as every week that passes reveals that bird flu is embedded in more ducks and chickens across a larger region of the globe than anyone thought possible. An estimated 120 million birds have already been culled in the Far East but the disease keeps returning, however much farmers try to eradicate it. By November 2005, it had returned to Thailand and infected a toddler and his grandmother. China, meanwhile, was just beginning to reveal the fact, long suspected by scientists, that poultry carry the disease in many of its regions, and that three human cases have been identified there.

In the autumn of 2005 when infected finches turned up in a quarantine facility near Essex, there were some alarmist newspaper headlines suggesting that the disease was in the UK, right now, in a way that was a dramatic threat to the human population. That is a very long way from the truth. However, others who feel that the whole issue is being over-hyped, blown up out of all proportion by the media looking for a new scare story, are off the mark as well.

In the words of Britain's chief medical officer Sir Liam Donaldson, a pandemic is a 'biological inevitability' and one that the World Health Organization has classified as the globe's most serious health challenge. Apart from the financial damage it could do – a severe pandemic could wipe out 2 per cent of the global economy – the mortality rates could be extremely high. The continent of Africa, for example, already crippled by the burden of HIV and malaria, couldn't begin to cope with a pandemic of a respiratory disease like influenza.

In Britain, there are two major dangers that need to be thought of in separate boxes. First, there is a risk that H5N1 will arrive here in birds quite soon, simply because all kinds of waterfowl migrate from the east into the UK over the winter months. The country has an excellent surveillance system set up to detect the first cases, so British vets would soon know if it was here. If it does arrive, there are serious implications for free-range poultry farmers and for those who run our bird reserves – but this hasn't happened yet.

The much greater worry is that a human influenza pandemic is overdue, and the dice are heavily loaded in favour of that pandemic being caused by H5N1. A reservoir of this disease probably lies in more than half a billion birds in the Far East, and it would take only a few genetic changes for it to move into people. There is very widespread pessimism among scientists that we would not have any real chance of containing the virus by extinguishing the first spark as soon as it appears. Mathematical modelling suggests the disease could be in the UK within two to four weeks of first being detected in Southeast Asia.

I began to want to write this book at the end of 2004 when I realized that although the UK government was taking the threat very seriously, they were not communicating the full extent of the danger to the public, and appeared to have no desire to tell us what to do about it. It is the nature of politics that you don't go around alarming people unless you've also got a very reassuring message to give them. 'Alertness, not panic' is a key phrase heard in the corridors of Westminster at the moment – but it is hard to be alert if no one is giving you all the information you need.

At about that time, I was researching bird flu for what would be my first article on the subject for the *Observer*. One of the government's special advisers realized I knew something about their emergency plan and asked me not to write about it. 'It's not very helpful to us,' he said. 'We still have some work to do on this. We don't want to create a public panic.'

There is this peculiarly British attitude that if you tell the public about risks, they will not be mature enough to weigh up the facts, or assess the information. But it was quite clearly the public pressure to address the threat that forced ministers into stockpiling antiviral medication at an early stage in 2005, and this has left the UK in a better position than most to face a pandemic.

As Professor Peter Openshaw, a highly respected respiratory infections expert, makes clear in his foreword, we live in an age when it is no longer possible to filter the news by central command. The public has a massive amount of knowledge and science available at the click of an Internet server. AOL, for example, reports that bird flu is consistently in its top ten hits.

Amid all the panic and uncertainty, we are not being told what we personally can do to prepare for the threat. By that, I don't mean building up our own armoury of pills and masks – that strategy would be quite limited in its success. It's about looking at many different aspects of your life, both at work and at home, and knowing what steps to take if you do catch the flu.

This book tries to address three main themes. First, it explains what the bird flu virus is, how it works, and why H5N1 might become a pandemic. Second, it looks at the way bird flu swept through countries like Thailand and shows how some of the poorest nations were left attempting to suppress the infection without proper resources or help; belatedly the world is trying to make up for those early mistakes. Third, and probably most importantly, it looks at how we would be affected both at work and at home during a pandemic, and what we can all do to help ourselves.

What is becoming increasingly clear to me, and many of the doctors I speak to, is that it will be crucial to learn how to manage the symptoms and protect yourself, as much as possible, from exposure to the virus when it does arrive. There is no magic cure, no invisibility cloak that you can don to prevent yourself from getting pandemic flu. But forewarned is indeed forearmed when it comes to something as contagious as influenza. By preparing your home with a few basic measures, and by teaching your children simple handwashing techniques, you can do something to cut back on the risk of infection. Do masks work? What should you do when someone next to you sneezes? And if your children or other family members become infected, how can you best look after them?

These are questions that I couldn't answer for myself but by talking to many experts around the world, I now have a much clearer idea of what will work and what won't – and I've tried to give the answers as clearly as possible in the later chapters.

One of the most important measures will be to stay at home if you develop any flu-like symptoms. Our impulse is to carry on working no matter what, to go to the chemist, or to the shops to stock up on food, but the single most important message has to be that if you are ill, you must not leave home.

There is another lesson for society that I suspect might be learned the hard way. Bird flu will test the humanity of every one of us in a way it hasn't been tested since World War II. Imagine for a minute that Britain is in its fourth week of a flu pandemic. The shops are running low on food, doctors' surgeries are besieged by patients desperate for anti-viral drugs, and the police are worried by the number of officers going down with flu symptoms. What would you do to help your elderly neighbour who lives across the road? You know she is there by herself; will you go over to her house and offer her some of your food? Would you invite her for a meal, not knowing whether she might be carrying the virus?

The impulse to care for one another, whether it is a neighbour or a sick relative, will be fundamental to how we ride this storm. We have seen acts of genuine courage and selflessness during the London bombings of 2005, but it remains to be seen how an entire community would behave in the midst of such a disease. If we prepare for the worst now, we will be in a slightly better position to care for others when the time comes.

I wanted this book to be both easily understandable yet detailed enough to give readers a full idea of how bird flu developed, and how we should respond to it. Further information can be accessed via the websites listed at the back of the book (see page 215). There is also a glossary of the scientific terms (see page 209) that I think we are going to hear a lot more about in the coming months. The Question and Answer section (see page 189) is there for readers who want to check something quickly, or who have a particular interest in one topic.

I hope you find the book of interest, and that instead of feeling scared by the thought of bird flu, you can read this and realize that governments around the world are finally responding to the threat by trying to share their expertise and investing in vaccines and healthcare. Above all, I hope it gives you some useful tips on how we can all prepare for a pandemic, calmly and without panic.

1 INFLUENZA, THE ULTIMATE MASTER OF DISGUISE

'I was panting, so tired, like I had been running for many kilometres non-stop, like I was going to stop breathing. The breath was so slight, it felt as if it could be gone any second.'

Pranom Thongchan — Bird flu survivor, Thailand

Influenza is a virus, a strange creature which is caught between the world of the living and the non-living. It floats in droplets in the air or sticks onto clothes, computers or skin, but it only really comes alive once it has infected another living form. Invasion is essential for its survival. Unlike bacteria, which are complex organisms that can reproduce by themselves, a virus is not self-sufficient. It exists to breed and can only do that by locking onto another organism and entering it, by stealth or force.

This highly elusive creature, evolved over many millions of years, is what we are up against in the fight against bird flu. Almost every day, newspapers and television bulletins are broadcasting new developments about the disease, and people are becoming more and more alarmed by the apparent ease with which it spreads. We have become used to the idea of a certain number of elderly people dying of flu each winter, but the infection we have seen in the Far East seems to be something entirely different, as it kills fit, healthy adults within days. What is it about this virus that makes it so lethal, and can the human body mount any defence against it?

The flu virus's single greatest asset is that it is airborne. Once the virus has invaded the cells lining your lungs, throat and nose, it sheds tiny particles which can be expelled at great speed in mucus when you sneeze, or in droplets of moisture from a cough or splutter. One study demonstrated that a viral particle can travel from one end of a train carriage to another at 80 miles an hour (128 km/hour), such is the force of the common sneeze. That is why covering the mouth and nose when you sneeze is far more than an issue of social etiquette; it is about preventing germs from escaping at high speed and infecting others near you.

The flu virus can also be carried on the skin. One common way in which you can become infected is if you shake hands with someone who is carrying the virus and then rub your eyes, nose or mouth with your hand. In fact, the particles can live for 48 hours on the surfaces of toys, doorknobs or computer keyboards – any hard surface will do. Disinfectant will kill them, and normal washing with soap and water would probably destroy most of the particles. Sunlight also destroys the germs, as does dry air. Even if there are particles on raw meat, once it is properly cooked the heat will have killed them.

Most of us have some natural immunity to the strains of flu that are usually circulating, but those with impaired immune systems or respiratory problems, such as asthma, are vulnerable and people with diabetes or heart disease can find their conditions exacerbated by a flu infection. There may be respiratory complications, such as bronchitis, or secondary infections such as ear problems, which are especially common in children. Pneumonia is one of the leading causes of death in patients with influenza. It develops when the lungs become inflamed by bacteria, such as *staphylococcus aureus*, because the tiny hairs (cilia) that normally protect the lungs from any dust, debris and bacteria are damaged by the virus. Antibiotics would be prescribed for pneumonia or other secondary bacterial infections, but they don't work against the flu itself, which is a virus.

In most northern hemisphere countries, seasonal flu lasts for between six and eight weeks each winter, often peaking in January. In the UK, around one in five people who becomes ill consults their GP, according to the Department of Health. When more than 200 new patients are consulting their GPs per week for every 100,000 of the population, the flu outbreak is said to have reached an epidemic level.

Flu would normally cause around as many as 12,000 deaths a year in the UK, but our immunization programme is helping to reduce the level of mortality. The flu vaccine is given each autumn to asthma sufferers, those aged 65 or over, residents in nursing homes or those with chronic problems such as heart disease, providing immunity against the major strains of flu that are expected to be in circulation that winter. However, it is always possible that a new strain emerges that they have not been immunized against – and the fear with bird flu is that if it leaps into humans, it would be a particularly powerful strain of flu against which we would have no ready-made vaccines, and no natural immunity.

'One study demonstrated that a viral particle can travel from one end of a train carriage to another at 80 miles an hour (128 km/hour), such is the force of the common sneeze.'

WHY BIRD FLU COULD CAUSE A PANDEMIC

So far, 130 human cases of bird flu – and 67 deaths – have been reported in Cambodia, China, Indonesia, Thailand and Vietnam since 2003. At the moment, it is actually extremely difficult for a human to catch the disease from a bird, and the great majority of those who have caught it have come into very close contact with ducks or hens. If it was easily transmitted, we would have seen hundreds of thousands of people fall ill by now, because there are many millions of ducks, hens and wild birds carrying the infection in Southeast Asia.

The bird flu virus can live in the droppings, saliva or nasal secretions of a bird. The wild birds who carry the virus, mostly waterfowl who fly between rivers and lakes, may fall ill or they may have no symptoms at all, but any droppings they leave behind at their stopping places can infect other birds.

The big worry now is that one particular strain of bird flu, known as H5N1, will become a human pathogen (disease-causing entity) and cause a flu pandemic. Until 1997, scientists didn't think it was possible for a bird flu virus to leap directly into humans, but now they know they were wrong.

It was back in 1933 that an enormous leap was made in the understanding of influenza. During a flu epidemic that year, Christopher Andrewes and Wilson Smith, scientists at the National Institute for Medical Research in London, inoculated ferrets with material taken from the throat of Andrewes himself while he was ill with a dose of human flu. Several days later the ferrets were sneezing and feverish, so the two men realized that the virus was able to spread from human to ferret, and then from ferret to ferret.

'At the moment, it is actually extremely difficult for a human to catch the disease from a bird, and the great majority of those who have caught it have come into very close contact with ducks or hens.'

Soon after, an even bigger breakthrough was made. An inoculated ferret sneezed in the face of a researcher and, two days later, he came down with the flu, proving that it could spread from animals to people. They had shown that a virus is capable of leaping between species. Two years later Wilson Smith discovered that the flu virus can be cultivated in chick embryos, a discovery that paved the way for vaccines to be created.

The great concern is that H5N1 bird flu will mutate to become a form which is easily transmissible from human to human. This has not happened yet, and it is impossible for anyone to say when it might happen, although experts very much fear that it will. Professor John Oxford, Professor of virology at Queen Mary's School of Medicine and Dentistry at the University of London, explained one possible scenario: 'If a child comes home from market carrying a chicken, and that chicken is then slaughtered in the back yard, it is possible that one of the family will breathe in the particles of virus from the bird. If that family member has a more common strain of flu which is around at the time, the H5N1 could mix its genes with the other form, and we could get a completely new form, against which we would have no immunity.

'This strain could evolve as it spread, acquiring new characteristics between people. It may, for example, become slightly less virulent because what matters to the virus is that the people it occupies don't die too quickly, but survive for long enough to pass it onto others. But it would still be a very powerful strain against which we have no defences.'

The human race has never been afflicted before with an H5N1 strain of flu and it is impossible to predict how lethal it might be, although our vulnerability would be high because we have no natural immunity to it. The fact that H5N1 has also spread between certain animals – tigers, peacocks, cats, pigs and several different species of birds – suggests it would be possible for transmission to become quite efficient from birds to humans.

H5N1 has been picked out as the flu subtype where a mutation into a fully 'humanized' strain is most likely to occur and cause a pandemic simply because the reservoir of disease is so great – there are just so many wild and domestic birds now harbouring the virus. So far it has proved to be a fairly lethal strain, despite the fact that it has not become a fully human-to-human disease yet. Those who have inhaled the bird flu virus have become ill very quickly. Once admitted to hospital, drugs have been administered and patients have been put on ventilators to aid their breathing, but they frequently die anyway.

The effect of the infection in humans can be quite devastating, as Dr Dominic Dwyer, a virologist and member of Australia's National Pandemic Planning Committee, explains: 'The virus gets into the lungs. The body makes a really strong immune response to it. The lungs fill up with fluid, with proteins, with cells that are all trying to get rid of the infection, but in fact what happens is the lungs fill up and the person can't breathe. They essentially die of respiratory failure. They can't breathe, they can't get enough oxygen in and that's it.'

In the cases seen in Vietnam and elsewhere, the disease is not confined to the respiratory tract. Back in February 2004, a report came through from Vietnam that a four-year-old boy and his nine-year-old sister had died from the brain disease encephalitis. According to a report for the *New England Journal of Medicine* by physicians in Ho Chi Minh City, the children were later found to have been infected with the H5N1 virus. During a postmortem examination, investigators found the virus in the cerebrospinal fluid, the blood, the throat and the gut of the children. Both had come into the hospital with severe diarrhoea but quickly deteriorated, suffering seizures, and then had fallen into a coma before they died.

'The lungs fill up with fluid, with proteins, with cells that are all trying to get rid of the infection, but in fact what happens is the lungs fill up and the person can't breathe. They essentially die of respiratory failure.'

Dr James D. Campbell, an influenza expert and an assistant professor of paediatrics at the University of Maryland School of Medicine, observed that encephalitis sometimes does occur with flu. 'What is unusual is that these cases of encephalitis occurred without respiratory symptoms,' he wrote in the *New England Journal of Medicine*. 'If it is true that this is a common way that infection with avian influenza presents, we will have to start looking for it in other than respiratory illnesses.'

If avian flu mutates to allow efficient human-to-human infection, it stands a good chance of becoming a pandemic, which is defined as an epidemic that has spread across more than one continent. Pandemics have a much higher 'attack rate' than normal flu, with up to 20 or 30 per cent of the population at large, and 50 per cent of children catching the infection. Some pandemics have a relatively high mortality rate, like the 1918 Spanish flu pandemic described in Chapter 2, which killed 2.5 per cent of all those who caught it, while others have a lower rate, like the 0.37 per cent who died in the 1957 flu outbreak.

It's not always the elderly who are worst affected in a flu pandemic – sometimes younger age groups are more at risk. The race is on for scientists to find out as much as they can about H5N1 and detect any mutations that make it a human-to-human virus as soon as possible. At least then they will know exactly what it is they are fighting.

WHAT IS A VIRUS?

Viruses have been around for several million years, but despite the enormous impact they have had on mankind they are still not fully understood. It was in 1933 that the scientists in London first isolated flu as a virus, and ten years later they were able to gaze at the enemy for the first time, thanks to the invention of the electron

'In many ways [a virus is] the perfect form of bio-terrorism – simple yet devastating.'

microscope. During the last 30 years, new molecular technology has enabled them to disentangle the genes and understand more about how viruses defeat our immune systems. But they still hold many mysteries that have yet to be solved.

Over the millennia, viruses have found a niche on this planet. By getting into the gut of an animal, they can weaken it for long enough to give them time to replicate and spread to other creatures. Over time, the flu virus has adapted not simply to enter the guts of chickens and ducks but also to enter humans' throats and lungs. It is expelled at enormous speed via a cough or a sneeze, providing a method of transport between hosts. In many ways, it's the perfect form of bio-terrorism – simple yet devastating.

In humans, these tiny particles – you could fit 1 million of them on a human hair – are breathed in through the nose or the mouth and they travel down your airway into the lungs. When they are inside the body, a set of proteins latches onto the cells lining the lungs, and breaks into them by stealth. Once inside, the virus is able to make hundreds of copies of itself by hijacking a cell's own reproductive machinery. It spreads across to other cells, releasing more material and causing enormous destruction.

There are three families of flu viruses, categorized as A, B and C, depending on their molecular structure. They are known scientifically as 'orthomyxoviruses', part of the family that causes mumps and measles.

The C influenza viruses are the most harmless and most common, and cause nothing more than a cold and a high temperature. It is usually those belonging to the B family that give us our seasonal outbreaks of flu, and the variety of symptoms with which we are familiar. Type A influenza viruses, which are usually found in wild birds or other animals, have evolved over millions of years, but along very different genetic lines from the B and C viruses.

'Under an electron microscope you would see something that looks like a spiky pincushion. Inside its fatty coat is the virus's genetic material.'

Many different kinds of influenza A viruses, usually harmless, live in the guts of wild birds for a few days before they are excreted. It is when they get into domestic birds – or humans – that they can cause damage. They infect the gut, cause sickness, and normally kill the birds within three days. In human beings, it is usually the respiratory system that is attacked.

The peculiar characteristics of influenza A viruses allow them to infiltrate our body in a way that is unique. They are an average size for a virus at about 100 nanometers (one thousand-millionth of a metre) in diameter. Under an electron microscope you would see something that looks like a spiky pincushion. Inside its fatty coat is the virus's genetic material. Inside each influenza A virus there are eight gene segments wrapped up in protective strands of a chemical called ribonucleic acid, or RNA. Some viruses are made of RNA, while others – such as smallpox – are made of deoxyribonucleic acid (DNA).

The spikes sticking out of the pincushion are actually pieces of protein, and the two key ones which give the virus its destructive nature are neuraminidase (NA) and haemagglutinin (HA). You may hear a lot about these in coming months, because they are the chemicals which scientists need to target to beat the flu.

One reason why influenza A viruses are so lethal to humans is because haemagglutinin possesses an amazing ability to unlock the cells of the host animal it has entered. It does this by latching onto certain receptors which lie on the surface of the host's cells. The receptor, which is like an entry point, believes it is letting in some food or a hormone and doesn't recognize the enemy. In chickens, the HA protein, or enzyme, is skilful at opening the cells of the birds' intestines, but in humans, the virus binds to receptors which line the upper respiratory tract (the throat and the upper lungs).

Once it has managed to trick the cell into opening up, the virus enters covered in some of the host cell's own plasma membrane – disguised, in other words. The membrane dissolves as the acidity of the cell changes and the virus's own genetic material is released. It enters the nucleus of the host cell and commandeers that cell's own reproductive machinery in order to make many hundreds of copies of itself. Some will contain errors, because an RNA virus has no way of 'proofreading' a copy to check for mistakes. But it has served its main purpose, which is to reproduce.

In order to spread through the body, the NA protein is essential. It can slice through the newly made bit of virus so that it is freed from the host cell and free to spread to the rest of the body. It is this particular protein which is targeted by the drug Tamiflu, or oseltamivir, which is explained in more detail in Chapter 5.

THE UNFAITHFUL BLUEPRINT

Unlike a DNA virus, when an RNA virus replicates, it makes a series of tiny errors. The copy is unfaithful, rather like a pamphlet from a very poor printing press. Nucleotides, the subunits of RNA which are strung together in a long chain, may change as the virus replicates and spreads between cells. This is what is known in science as a mutation. Because the viruses replicate at great speed, these errors or mutations happen uncontrollably and very fast.

What would be the evolutionary purpose of an RNA virus

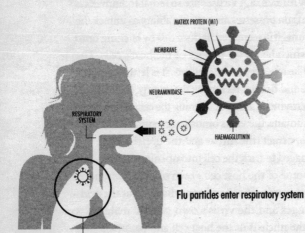

MATRIX PROTEIN (M1)

MEMBRANE

NEURAMINIDASE

RESPIRATORY SYSTEM

HAEMAGGLUTININ

1

Flu particles enter respiratory system

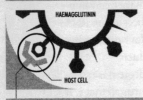

HAEMAGGLUTININ

HOST CELL

2

Haemagglutinin latches onto host cells in throat and upper lungs, and unlocks them. The host cell believes the virus to be useful, like a food or hormone

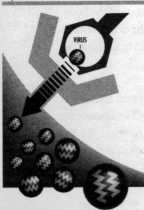

VIRUS

3

Virus enters the nucleus of the host cell, and hijacks that cell's own reproductive machinery in order to make hundreds of copies of itself

4

Virus spreads through the body causing possible coma or death

Infiltrating the body   The stages of flu infection

allowing errors every time it breeds? You might think that nature wouldn't favour any kind of organism that couldn't make faithful copies of its own genes. But the enormous benefit this frenzied mutation confers is that many strains of the virus will appear, and eventually one strain will emerge that is stronger, or more resistant, or more transmissible than all the rest. This is exactly what we see with flu every year, when the different strains 'compete' against one another to become the dominant infectious agent.

The constant 'shape-shifting' of the virus also means that it can constantly evade detection by an animal's immune system. With an influenza virus, this allows it to spread through the respiratory system before the body has a chance of defending itself. Antibodies are the chemicals produced by your bodies that are able to lock onto foreign bits of protein, known as antigens, and mark them out for destruction. With normal flu strains that have been circulating in the population for a while, our bodies recognize and destroy these antigens very quickly. But influenza A viruses are continuously changing the proteins that make up their outer coat, so that the immune system's memory cells have no way of 'remembering' them. Our antibodies have no recognition of the antigens, so it has to be learned, which takes time.

'...the enormous benefit this frenzied mutation confers is that many strains of the virus will appear, and eventually one strain will emerge that is stronger, or more resistant, or more transmissible than all the rest.'

If you are infected with a new strain of flu virus, your body will try to produce antibodies that will bind to that specific strain's antigen, or viral protein. Once it binds to it, it can stop the virus from infecting other cells. Those who have been infected will carry those antibodies in their blood and can be tested for them. But with a totally new strain, the antibodies might be produced by the body too late to mount an effective defence.

As Professor Peter Openshaw explains to me from his rooms at St Mary's Hospital in London, a flu virus's genetic make-up gives it a big advantage. 'DNA viruses are lumbering, sophisticated machines which carry their own coding with them. They are viruses like smallpox which contain hundreds of genes which control the host's immune responses. And then there are RNA viruses, which are lighter, evolve rapidly, much faster and produce a swarm of variants. The flu virus has a commando style rather than using the heavy machinery of the artillery. It will invade, wreck a cell and then leave the destruction behind quickly.'

What can our bodies do, faced with such an enemy? Our immune systems were never designed to cope with such fast and reckless invaders.

'What can our bodies do, faced with such an enemy? Our immune systems were never designed to cope with such fast and reckless invaders.'

VIRAL POSTCODES

Each flu virus belongs to a type – A, B or C – but then it also has a subtype, and these are named according to the classes of the neuraminidase (NA) or the haemagglutinin (HA) sticking out of it. There are sixteen different HA subtypes and nine different NA subtypes, all of which in different combinations can affect birds, but only some of which will infect humans.

In 2003, there was a serious outbreak of bird flu found in poultry in the Netherlands and, after tests, it was categorized as H7N7. This was because it was found to contain type 7 HA, and type 7 NA. It did infect people, but only mildly. The Dutch acted remarkably quickly and managed to stop it in its tracks before it mutated any further (see page 77).

Only certain influenza A subtypes – H1N1, H1N2 and H3N2 – generally circulate in the human population. Other subtypes are found most commonly in other animal species. H7N7 and H3N8 viruses, for example, cause illness in horses. The form of bird flu which scientists have been so concerned about ever since it emerged in Hong Kong in 1997 is known as H5N1.

Think of this number as a postcode. It gives scientists an idea of the kind of virus they are looking at, but not its exact address. Within this postcode, there are different variations of H5N1. Doctors will also label it as high pathogen (HP) or low pathogen (LP), describing its ability to cause either serious disease or only mild illness.

But there is yet another distinction which is necessary when classifying the viruses because they mutate so readily, and you have to be able to talk about different variants, which are called strains. When a sample is taken to the lab and grown in culture it is known as an 'isolate'; through the use of isolates, a virus's genetic code is studied.

And, to be even more accurate, there is yet another definition which a flu virus will be given, which is its 'genotype' – its special genetic make-up based on the various combinations of the eight separate gene segments it contains. The H5N1 virus has changed its genotype several times since it first emerged in Hong Kong in 1997. Between 1998 and 2001, many small changes to its genetic make-up occurred, and in 2002, some birds which died in a park in Hong Kong were found to have a particular genetic make-up, which was given the name of Genotype Z, or GenZ for short. This currently appears to be the dominant form of H5N1.

> *'The form of bird flu which scientists have been so concerned about ever since it emerged in Hong Kong in 1997 is known as H5N1.'*

But the virus has evolved further as it spread across nine different Asian nations. Within the genotype of GenZ, there are now two different forms known as 'clades', a scientific term for a group of organisms which have one common ancestor, and therefore have similar features. It comes from the Greek word *klados*, meaning branch, and it's a useful way of seeing how the virus can branch out to have different characteristics.

Flu viruses are classified according to the following:

- *type*
- *subtype*
- *strain*
- *genotype*
- *clade*

The world now has Clade One and Clade Two H5N1. The former is the strain which is dominant in Vietnam, Thailand, Laos and Cambodia, and the latter has been found in China, Japan, Korea and Indonesia. Clade Two is also the one that has come to Europe, and infected birds in Greece, Turkey, Romania and Croatia.

There are two ways in which an influenza A virus can jump from species to species, known to virologists as 'drift or shift'.

• When subtypes of a virus from different species, such as a bird and a human, trade and merge their genes, the result is an entirely new strain. This is known as 'antigenic shift', because the antigen – the particular protein the flu is targeting – has changed and the result is a new subtype.

• With antigenic drift, there are small but important changes that happen to the genetic material in the virus over time as it goes on replicating, and the virus gradually adapts to become one that can easily infect humans.

It is the shifting, or reassorting of the genetic material, which has resulted in lethal pandemics in the past. By mixing with a human influenza virus in the way Professor John Oxford suggested, the disease could become easily transmissible between people for long enough to allow it to spread far and wide.

We are still in the process of discovering more about it, according to Dr Alan Hay, director of the World Influenza Centre in north London. This centre, established at the National Institute for Medical Research just after World War II, has been at the forefront of global efforts to detect the emergence of new and potentially lethal strains. It is one of four World Health Organization (WHO) collaborating centres for reference and research on influenza, and every year it makes recommendations about which new strains should go into the preparation of that year's flu vaccine.

'What we have seen is the persistence of this genotype [GenZ] to become the predominant one, but we have seen also these two clades emerge in different countries,' explained Dr Hay. 'It is hard to say which clade might be worse for human health. We don't know whether one of them could infect us more readily than the other. But at the moment, the greatest risk is what might come out of Southeast Asia.'

2 LESSONS FROM PANDEMICS OF THE LAST CENTURY

'From the point of view of humankind, the main characteristic of influenza is its ability to spread by aerosol [dispersal of particles through the air]. Other infections like polio spread in the water, so you can decontaminate it. With HIV, you can stop it by not having unprotected sex. But you can't stop breathing. There's nothing you can do, unless you are going to live like a hermit in the desert. As we come more into contact with each other, as cities grow, viruses have this fantastic opportunity – and they tend to take it.'

Professor John Oxford   Professor of Virology, University of London

The former British colony of Hong Kong, known for its wealth, its towering edifices and a proud trading history, doesn't panic easily. But back in December 1997, fear spread across the province as the first reports began to emerge of a lethal virus that was killing people within two or three days of infection.

The first appearance of this deadly flu appears to have been in May 1997. A three-year-old boy was brought into hospital with a cough and a slight fever. Two days later, his symptoms had worsened and he was having breathing difficulties as well as suffering a severe headache and a sore throat. The doctors pumped him full of antibiotics and put him on a ventilator to ease his breathing, but within six days of admission he had died.

Seven months later, a 51-year-old dentist in Hong Kong fell ill and died. Within a short space of time, he was followed by sixteen others, all of whom showed alarmingly similar symptoms. The infectious diseases experts, realizing that they were dealing with something unusual, had the foresight to call laboratories in both the USA and Holland to try and identify what appeared to be a new kind of virus.

It soon became apparent that there was one factor the human cases all had in common – they had recently visited one of Hong Kong's live-poultry markets, the centres where many residents go to buy their fresh meat and eggs.

Albert Osterhaus, a global authority on bird flu and a leading 'virus-hunter' who runs the virology department of the Erasmus Medical Center in Rotterdam in the Netherlands, was sent one of the samples. Sitting in the garden of an Oxford college in September 2005, he recounted to me the drama of that December. 'We tested this virus with the normal human reagents, looking for something common, but they all came back negative. As a team, we thought this was strange.'

They managed to work out the virus's genotype by sequencing it, and this showed it was H5N1 – a form of avian influenza. Dr Osterhaus shook his head as he recalled the events. 'It didn't make sense because this isn't supposed to happen. A disease leaping from birds to humans – it was against all the rules.'

The lab results in Rotterdam, which were confirmed by experts at the US Center for Disease Control and Prevention in Atlanta, Georgia, showed that the human samples matched a strain of a virus that had raged through poultry farms in Hong Kong's New Territories back in April 1997. The unthinkable had happened. Until this point in history, no one had imagined that birds could transmit their viral infections directly to human beings. The genetic leap was said to be too great for this feat to occur – before that they thought that pigs acted as a mixing vessel between birds and humans – but here, in Hong Kong, the evidence was staring them in the face. This was the first time scientists had firm evidence that a bird flu virus could make the jump directly into humans.

Panic swept through the colony. The public understood that in a densely populated city, there would be little protection against an epidemic. Thousands turned up at the hospitals, worried that their coughs might be a symptom of something worse. Many demanded tests, but there wasn't any way of making a rapid diagnosis. Hospital staff started to wear masks for fear of contamination. The health authorities begged the government to act quickly. They did – they took the only course of action open to them, and in doing so probably averted a worldwide pandemic.

HOW HONG KONG SAVED THE WORLD

One of the world's largest-ever bird culls took place on 29 December 1997. Within the space of three days, nearly 1.5 million chickens, geese, pigeons, ducks and quail were destroyed. The bodies were buried in mass graves on landfill sites. No one had ever attempted such a huge cull in such a short timespan.

'The unthinkable had happened. Until this point in history, no one had imagined that birds could transmit their viral infections directly to human beings. The genetic leap was said to be too great for this feat to occur...'

At the Hung Hom market in Kowloon, Hong Kong, officials wearing white coats and black rubber boots were sent in to carry out the slaughter. It was not a pretty sight. They either cut the birds' throats or gassed them with carbon dioxide. Some of the market traders insisted they killed the birds themselves, to prevent prolonged suffering. One trader named Chung San rolled up his sleeves, grabbed a chicken and cut its throat, blood splashing over his bare arms. 'I don't need any protection,' he declared stoically. 'I've already been to see the doctor and he says I'm fine.'

More than a thousand workers were drafted in to help with the cull. Some 900 shopkeepers and market-stallholders, and nearly 200 farmers watched all their livestock being slaughtered. Even the stray dogs roaming around the area were put down in case they might harbour the virus. Afterwards, the blood was hosed away and the entire area was sprayed with disinfectant.

One of the remarkable things about Hong Kong is the way its resilient population pull together in an emergency. The compensation payments were not high for those like Chung San who lost their livelihood, but traders knew that confidence in poultry had to be restored. It was much the same attitude that prevailed in Britain during the foot-and-mouth disease crisis, when farmers realized that they would have to cull thousands of cows in order to eradicate the disease and restore the public's trust in beef. Even though cooked chicken carries no risk, because the virus is destroyed once it is heated properly, the entire state of Hong Kong had stopped eating poultry and the airlines flying out of the city's international airport had pulled it from their menus.

Hong Kong's troubles were far from over, despite their fast reaction. In 2001, another deadly strain of H5N1 was found in the markets, and again, the killing of poultry was essential. At the beginning of 2002, the flu re-emerged. It seemed as if the Territories would never be free of it. The problem was that the virus was regularly crossing the border into Hong Kong from neighbouring Guangdong Province in southern China, a region with a peasant economy where the people live alongside their ducks and hens. Many birds were being transported across the border, for consumption and also for breeding, so the virus kept re-appearing in Hong Kong.

In all, Hong Kong had eighteen recorded human cases of bird flu in 1997, and six of them died. In 2003, there were two further deaths. A family of five – mother, father, two sisters and a brother – visited Fujian in China. The younger of the sisters died while in China, but the cause of her death was never established. Once back in Hong Kong, the nine-year-old boy and his father fell ill and were admitted to the Princess Margaret Hospital, where it was found that they were infected with the H5N1 virus. The boy had a low fever, cough and a runny nose on 9 February when he came in, but three days later, X-rays showed that his lungs were seriously infected. His father had different symptoms, including nosebleeds, nausea and abdominal pain. None of the treatment they gave the father was enough to save him and he died six days after being admitted to hospital. The boy, however, survived.

THE ARRIVAL OF A NEW BIOLOGICAL KILLER

As if Hong Kong had not been through enough, in the spring of 2003 a different kind of biological entity afflicted the state. Several people who had recently travelled into mainland China turned up in Hong Kong that March with severe pneumonia. Health officials assumed it was the H5N1 virus again, and began to look urgently for the source of the outbreak. However, Malik Peiris, a renowned Sri Lankan virologist who is known in his field as a quiet and unassuming man, suspected that this might be something other than bird flu.

'At the end of January [2003] we heard these stories coming out of Guangdong about unusual pneumonia that was kicking around. Our first thought was maybe this [bird flu] virus had gone human. That was what we really set out to catch.'

Back in 1995, Professor Peiris had assembled a first-class team of virologists at Hong Kong University and he led them with admirable calmness through the bird flu outbreak of 1997. He recounts their reaction when they became aware of the 2003 virus: 'At the end of January [2003] we heard these stories coming out of Guangdong about unusual pneumonia that was kicking around. Our first thought was maybe this [bird flu] virus had gone human. That was what we really set out to catch.'

Both Professor Peiris and the US Center for Disease Control and Prevention (CDC) in Atlanta started to test viral samples taken from patients, by adding the specimens to normal cell cultures in a laboratory and seeing if they changed. But nothing was happening. The Hong Kong team then started trying out more unusual cell types, and one of them – kidney cells taken from a monkey – showed results. The virus turned out to be a coronavirus (a microbe with a different kind of genetic make-up to the flu virus), which had been Peiris's hunch all along, and it was given the name SARS (severe acute respiratory syndrome).

'Let's get this straight – Malik is the one who discovered SARS, not the CDC, not someone else. They were all behind,' said Dr Robert Webster, one of the world's most renowned avian influenza experts. 'We all thought it was bird flu. He is the one that identified SARS.'

That early diagnosis helped the world to understand what it was dealing with. When it spread to Canada, clinicians there were able to test for it and to take extremely rigorous infection control measures. Despite the panic, it turned out that SARS was not as easily transmissible as was initially thought, although it was still a lethal virus. It killed 800 out of the 8,500 people it infected, but the world had a narrow escape because the virus had not managed to turn itself into a microbe capable of spreading easily and quickly between humans.

THE LEAP BETWEEN SPECIES

SARS provided the world with a clear warning of what animal diseases can do to the human race if they manage to leap between species. Since the beginning of civilization, humans and animals have been living in the same quarters as one another, and many of the infections that plague us have come directly as a result of this domestic arrangement. Measles is thought to originate from cattle, as is tuberculosis. Whooping cough probably comes from pigs and ducks, and we can thank rodents for many terrible diseases such as Lassa fever. At the time of SARS, civet cats and ferrets that are sold in China's markets were blamed for the disease, but it is now thought that it actually originated in wild bats in China.

Professor Peiris believes that pig farms could provide the new launchpad for a human pandemic. In June 2005, he told a conference of animal experts: 'We have a virus that is inefficiently crossing to humans. But, as with SARS, if you leave this situation to continue for long enough, it is possible that virus may adapt to efficient human-to-human transmission.' As pigs are already carrying another human virus, known as H3N2, a ready opportunity exists for crossover, he believes. 'Obviously you have this setting where pigs and poultry are next to each other and you clearly have an opportunity for H5NI to cross into pigs who might be carrying the H3N2 virus.' Today chickens, tomorrow pigs – will humans be next?

Speaking to me from his lab in Hong Kong, he explained why he feels that the struggle to keep H5N1 under control in birds is one that will be long and hard. 'I think we reacted very quickly in 1997 but I think what is even more commendable is that since then we have been able to maintain very high surveillance levels. Even after 1997, it kept on coming back but because Hong Kong had this high level of detection it was picked up very early and then, over the next few years, we strengthened our defences. Now the message is – keep Hong Kong free. We have constant surveillance and we have others measures in live bird markets designed to pick it up. Others have followed suit. South Korea and Japan have been affected but because they picked it up at an early stage, they were able to control it.'

'In the past, pandemics have announced themselves with a sudden explosion of cases which took the world by surprise. This time, we have been given a clear warning.'

Far more research is needed into why the virus has managed to infect some people and not others, he added. 'We are still trying to understand why it causes such severe disease in humans.' But he does not think the risks have been overstated by scientists. 'I think the concern about a pandemic is justified. It's not one of those things anyone can predict with certainty. But with the best will in the world, it's quite difficult to do the proper surveillance because ducks can carry it but also be asymptomatic. That means that sometimes, the disease is invisible to us.'

Dr Lee Jong-Wook, director-general of the World Health Organization, echoes his concerns. 'In the past, pandemics have announced themselves with a sudden explosion of cases which took the world by surprise. This time, we have been given a clear warning.'

THE SPANISH FLU OUTBREAK OF 1918–19

History tells us much of what we need to know about the diseases of the future. The reason why Malik Peiris and others knew that bird flu could be bad news was because they were familiar with the literature of past pandemics. *Pandemos* is a Greek word meaning 'across the people'. In medical terminology, 'pandemic' signifies the worldwide spread of a disease, with outbreaks occurring in many countries either simultaneously or shortly after one another, and in most regions of the world.

Throughout history, influenza pandemics have swept across the globe causing a devastating number of deaths and bringing social and economic devastation in their wake. Three pandemics have occurred in the past century – the so-called 'Spanish flu' outbreak of 1918–19, the Asian flu of 1957–8 and the Hong Kong flu of 1968–9 – but by far the most severe of these was the 1918–19 pandemic. Given the name Spanish flu because news of the outbreak was freely reported in Spain, which was not involved in the war,

'In the days before long-haul travel and cheap flights, Spanish flu still managed to traverse the globe thanks to the boats that were ferrying soldiers across continents.'

the disease had a mortality rate of around 2.5 per cent (the percentage of those infected who died of the virus), which is far, far higher than any other recorded pandemic and higher than that of most infectious diseases. In those days, there were no vaccines or drugs to offer patients; Epsom salts was the recommended treatment. Old black and white photographs show London policemen holding handkerchiefs to their faces, in an attempt to stop themselves breathing in the germs that were affecting so much of the country.

John Oxford, Professor of Virology at Queen Mary's School of Medicine and Dentistry at the University of London, has devoted much of his career to tracking down the origins of the 1918 pandemic. He believes that it came from the chickens that were kept in the British army camps along the Western front. In particular, he links it to the base at Étaples where, in the winter of 1916, hundreds of soldiers went down with what was termed at the time 'purulent bronchitis' but looks now to have been classic influenza. As more than 1 million soldiers passed through this base between 1916 and 1918, it would have provided a perfect transmission route for the disease.

In the days before long-haul travel and cheap flights, Spanish flu still managed to traverse the globe thanks to the boats that were ferrying soldiers across continents. A military camp was the ideal setting for rapid transmission and it spread like wildfire through camps in the US, but because it was the middle of wartime not much attention was initially paid to it. Then there was a second wave of the pandemic, when it was brought back into the US from Europe at the end of 1918, travelling through ports that were busy with shipments of war machinery and supplies. Armistice Day on 11 November, 1918, was a disastrous event in public health terms, because there were large gatherings in many cities, giving the infection a perfect opportunity to take hold.

'An American skipping rhyme of 1918:
I had a little bird
Its name was Enza
I opened the window
And in-flu-enza.'

The effects of the contagion were staggering. It was so bad that when it hit America people thought it was a plague that had been deliberately manufactured by the Germans and secretly released into their homeland via a submarine. Others, more rationally, worried that it might be an outbreak of meningitis.

The virulence of the infection was frightening, with some victims dying within two to three days of infection. They suffered piercing headaches and fever, often followed by pneumonia and other complications. Some of the victims' faces turned blue as they were slowly drowning in their own lung fluid. It mainly affected healthy young adults between the ages of 20 and 40 – actually, it now seems that as many as 99 per cent of the victims were under 65. The fact that their immune system was robust and mounted such a strong defence against viral attack may have meant that their lung tissue broke down more quickly, and left them prey to complications.

The disease decimated the troops who were being sent abroad

to fight, or who languished in military camps. Of the American soldiers who died in Europe, half of them perished from influenza rather than enemy action. One doctor at an army camp near Boston wrote in September 1918 about the speed of the contagion. 'It is only a matter of a few hours until death comes, and it is simply a struggle for air until they suffocate. It is horrible.'

Professor David Killingray, a historian at Goldsmith's College in London, comments: 'Countries were not really prepared. They did not know it was a virus which was causing all the deaths, and instead concentrated on bacteria. Vaccines were developed, but it was a shotgun approach. People were pumped full of lots of things, which probably did more harm than good.'

'The streets of London were deserted. Schools were closed and public gatherings were banned.'

In every country that was affected, shops and businesses were closed for the three months that it lasted. The streets of London were deserted. Schools were closed and public gatherings were banned. In one American town, shaking hands was outlawed. Communities did recover, though, and when the second wave of the pandemic came, many people had immunity from having been infected – and survived – the first time round.

Altogether it is estimated that one fifth of the population of the world was infected by this devastating disease, and between 20 and 40 million died worldwide – although lack of data from Africa makes it difficult to quantify the real death toll, and the true figure could even be as high as 80 million.

- Around 23 per cent of the British population developed influenza, and around 250,000 died.

- In America, it infected 28 per cent of citizens and killed an estimated 675,000 people, ten times as many as died in World War I. It was so severe that the average lifespan in the US fell by ten years.

- Australia was hit by the infection a year after everyone else, but it still caused 11,500 deaths.

- Around 400,000 people died in France.
- It is estimated that 14 per cent of Fijians died within the space of two weeks when it struck their island and in Western Samoa, as many as 22 per cent of the population died.
- The countries which were worst affected were India, where up to 17 million people perished, and sub-Saharan Africa, where deaths numbered between 1.5 and 2 million (possibly many, many more).

WHAT WAS THE 1918 VIRUS?

So what exactly was the virus that caused such mass fatalities? The unravelling of the virus's code and the recreation of that strain is one of the great scientific stories of the last decade. We will never know her real name, but the body of 'Lucy', a young Inuit woman frozen in the permafrost of Alaska, told scientists more about the terrible pandemic of 1918 than they ever dared to believe they might discover.

'Lucy' had died in Brevig, Alaska, and had been buried in a mass grave in the permafrost. With the permission of local people, her grave was dug up in the 1990s and her frozen lung tissue was extracted by a retired pathologist who sent it to Dr Jeffery Taubenberger, chief of the molecular pathology department at the Armed Forces Institute of Pathology in Washington.

His institute had a warehouse containing tissue from old autopsies. There, Dr Taubenberger was able to find some tissue from two solders who had died of the Spanish flu of 1918 – tiny snips of lung soaked in formalin and encased in small blocks of wax. No one had touched them for nearly 80 years when he decided to examine them in 1995.

It took almost a year to put everything together, using the lung tissue from the Inuit woman, the soldiers and some other samples that had been preserved in strange ways over the years. During this time, the team published findings about the sequences of five of the eight genes and then, in October 1995, they published the last three.

After they had read the complete genetic code of the whole

virus, an H1N1 subtype, they were able to rebuild it from scratch. They did so in a laboratory so secure that the handful of scientists allowed in had to pass through retina scanners to prove their identity.

At the same time, some other American researchers were working on the virus. They infected mice and some tissue from human lungs to see if the virus would remain lethal if they switched some of its genes with genes from today's normal flu viruses. What they found is that even tiny substitutions of genetic material meant that the virus could no longer replicate in the animals, or attach itself to the lung cells.

Through his painstaking efforts, Dr Taubenberger established that instead of the virus mixing with a human flu strain through reassortment (see page 34), it adapted and leapt into people. It wasn't just one or two genes that changed, it was small mutations in all eight genes. 'I didn't expect it to be as lethal as it was,' he told the journal *Nature* in October 1995. His research showed that just a few tiny mutations in the genetic make-up of a virus can turn it into something extremely dangerous. This detective work was not just a technical feat; it also shed light on what the future might hold for us.

THE ASIAN FLU EPIDEMIC OF 1957–8

In May 1957 an epidemic of influenza was reported in Hong Kong, and epidemiologists agreed that the virus had first emerged in China earlier that year. This new strain spread rapidly to Japan, the Philippines, Malaysia and Indonesia and by June there were reports of infected passengers and crew on board ships that had stopped at Southeast Asian ports. The virus travelled across the world, in both an easterly and a westerly direction, and ports were generally the first cities to be affected in each country, indicating that the international shipping trade was the main vehicle by which it was being spread.

This flu epidemic was a much milder one than the Spanish flu 40 years earlier, but the brunt of the disease fell on the young (those between five and fourteen years old), and in 1957 up to half of all British schoolchildren were infected. The young seemed to have no natural immunity, but they mostly managed to fight it off and the majority of those who died were over the age of 55.

Unlike 1918, an animal virus had not leapt directly into people. Instead, there was reassortment when a human flu strain mixed with an avian one to present a new form. The World Health Organization, set up by the United Nations after World War II, was able to give countries an early warning that an outbreak was imminent when the virus started spreading across Southeast Asia. The strain of the virus – H2N2 – was quickly identified thanks to new scientific advances and a vaccine was made which saved the lives of thousands of people.

The virus arrived in the US quietly, with a series of small outbreaks over the summer of 1957. When American children went back to school in the autumn, they spread the disease in classrooms and brought it home to their families. Infection rates were highest among schoolchildren, young adults and pregnant women but, as elsewhere, the elderly had the highest death rates. Altogether nearly 70,000 Americans died, around 0.37 per cent of those who caught the infection.

'...ports were generally the first cities to be affected in each country, indicating that the international shipping trade was the main vehicle by which it was being spread.'

In Britain, the advent of the NHS and an integrated public health system also made an enormous difference; people were able to see a family doctor without worrying about how they were going to pay the bill. But it did have an enormous impact on the hospitals, which could barely cope. In some areas, up to one third of nurses were absent at the peak of the outbreak in the autumn of that year, because there were no anti-viral drugs available that would protect staff. They also ran out of beds when 30,000 more cases of acute respiratory infection were admitted to hospitals than would have been normal for the time of year. But the outbreak was fairly short-lived, and despite the fact that the young were most affected, nearly all schools had returned to normal four weeks after the first case. More than

30,000 deaths were recorded in England and Wales, but only 6,716 were attributed to the virus alone while the rest had secondary contributing factors.

By December 1957, the worst seemed to be over but in January and February 1958, a second wave of infection emerged. It is thought that 20,000 died in France from the 1957 pandemic, and the mortality rate in Australia was up to five times higher than in normal years. But the estimated global death toll of around 2 million was merciful in comparison to the tens of millions who had perished in 1918–19.

THE HONG KONG FLU OF 1968–9

This strain – H2N2 mixed with a human flu – was first isolated in July 1968 but it took a year to spread around the world, from Hong Kong through to Bangkok, Bombay, Washington, Rome, Lagos and Sao Paulo before it reached Sydney 342 days later.

In the US, the pandemic didn't gain momentum until December 1968, around the school holidays, and this meant that the rate of illness among schoolchildren and their families wasn't so high. In the UK, a strange pattern was seen. It was first detected in August 1968 and caused small community outbreaks that December, but the full epidemic in the UK came a year later. It is easy to assume that flu is a winter disease, but outbreaks can appear at any time of the year, not just in the traditional winter months.

This virus was a less dramatic 'shift' in genetic terms than the Asian flu of 1957–8, and was milder. Similarities to the Asian flu meant that many people had some immunity, so the death toll wasn't as high as it might have been. Also, improved medical care and antibiotics to deal with secondary infections helped to save many patients. Around 750,000 deaths were recorded globally, most of them among the elderly. In Britain there were 78,000 deaths, both from the flu and its complications such as pneumonia and bronchitis. In the US, many caught it but the death rate was less than half the previous pandemic's toll, with some 33,000 fatalities recorded.

However, mathematical modelling carried out by John Hopkins University in Baltimore, Maryland, suggests that a 21st-century pandemic would travel round the world much more quickly than Hong Kong flu did. The popularity of long-haul travel and the fact that so many people now live in cities could mean that it would take just 180 days for a virus to spread globally – half the time it took in 1968–9.

What the world has been given over the last 90 years is three clear warnings about how influenza can spread, quickly and effectively, around the globe. The fact that the last three pandemics happened in an age when there were no fast, cheap flights shows that flu will spread, no matter how hard you try to contain it.

Each pandemic has a different pattern. The virus will cause a set of symptoms which characterize it, and it will affect a particular age range, but this cannot be predicted before the event. If bird flu mutates into a human disease, capable of spreading quickly, it will have its own 'signature' and the best we can hope for is that this will be quickly identified by clinicians, who can alert doctors around the world about what to look out for.

'The popularity of long-haul travel and the fact that so many people now live in cities could mean that it would take just 180 days for a virus to spread globally – half the time it took in 1968–9.'

Hong Kong has shown us that with a very high level of surveillance and monitoring, it is possible to set up an 'early warning system' and detect the earliest cases of bird flu, before it has had a chance to infect many people – and particularly before the virus has had a chance to mutate further into a fully 'humanized' form of the disease, capable of infecting millions. We must learn the lessons from the past in order to understand how vigilant we need to be in the future.

3 THE KILLER IN THE RICE PADDIES

> '*This virus is already entrenched in Asia. It seems quite versatile and resilient – cunning in a way. If you look at the genetic information compared with five years ago, it has already changed and adapted. We have to do something urgently to prevent serious consequences – I mean a human pandemic.*'

Dr Shigeru Omi   World Health Organization Regional Director for the Western Pacific

Since the first outbreak of bird flu in Hong Kong in 1997, the world had been playing a waiting game. Where and how would the virus re-emerge? Experts had little doubt that it would return because these viruses are capable of lying low for years in the wild duck population. When it did re-emerge, it struck swiftly and with terrible consequences.

All over Southeast Asia, there are lots of regions where people live close together in smallholdings, with ducks, hens and other birds roaming about freely. They share communal ponds and outdoor slaughterhouses with their neighbours. It was communities like these that would prove to be the perfect breeding ground for the bird flu virus. But unlike those in Hong Kong, some health authorities didn't act swiftly enough to extinguish the latest outbreak. Whether for political reasons, lack of resources or insufficient expertise, their procrastination was to have dire consequences for human health.

THE WEDDING FEAST, JANUARY 2004

It is a sad irony that family gatherings can end up killing the loved ones who came together to celebrate. In January 2004, 31-year-old teacher Ngo Le Hung was preparing for his wedding feast. He bought a live chicken in the local market in his home town, which is surrounded by the rice paddies of the Red River delta of northern Vietnam. The chicken he chose was killed in his presence then slowly cooked with herbs. The whole family shared it at his wedding.

A few days later, Ngo Le Hung started to feel very ill. His muscles ached badly and a band of pain tightened round his head. Within 24 hours he had succumbed to the virus and collapsed. Six days after being admitted to hospital he died, and his bride Phong Thi Ngo Anh found herself a widow. Within the space of one week, his two sisters, Le Hong (30) and Le Hanh (23) had been struck down by bird flu, and they also died.

The deaths of three family members had ramifications far beyond the grief of the family and their friends. The news was greeted with consternation by international health experts, who feared that that this might be the first sign that the virus had mutated and become a human pathogen, capable of spreading not just from bird to human, but from human to human. Six years after the swift and decisive action taken by the Hong Kong authorities, the virus had made its dramatic re-appearance, and this time it appeared to be in the wetlands of northern Vietnam.

The Vietnamese ministry of health, faced with the prospect of enormous human suffering as well as drastic economic loss, called on experts from the World Health Organization (WHO) in Geneva to come to Hanoi and start investigating what had happened to Ngo Le Hung and his sisters. Scientists from the WHO and also the UN's Food and Agriculture Organization collected whatever serum samples they could from the victims and their families. Ngo Le Hung had already been cremated so there was no tissue available to study the virus that had killed him, but samples were taken from his sisters' bodies. These were flown out the same day to laboratories around the world for testing, using a technique known as Polymerase Chain Reaction (PCR), which is a way of looking at the genetic make-up of the virus.

For Dr Pham Van Diu, head of preventive medicine in Thai Binh, the town closest to where the family died, the five days he spent waiting for the results to come through were unbearable. But then, he felt enormous relief when the test results came back. They showed that the virus that had killed the three siblings was not a new human strain, but that they had all caught the H5N1 virus from being present at the slaughter of the chicken for the feast. The world could breathe a sigh of relief; the antigenic shift that everyone so dreaded had not yet taken place.

'It was hard for virologists and health experts from outside Vietnam to keep track of the virus during this period, because they were not allowed free access to samples from either the people or the birds.'

Communist-controlled northern Vietnam had just started to build up a tourist trade after years of poverty following the wars, and was not as rich as its neighbours. Although Hanoi has Western shops, restaurants and hotels, many of the villages out in the hinterland still operate as peasant economies and their poultry is essential to them for eggs and meat. Now they were being told that millions of chickens, ducks and birds had to be slaughtered to prevent the bird flu virus from spreading.

It was hard for virologists and health experts from outside Vietnam to keep track of the virus during this period, because they were not allowed free access to samples from either the people or the birds. How rigorous was the cull and over how wide an area? Maybe they dragged their feet, reluctant to deal with an issue that could have such a huge economic impact. Maybe they didn't have enough resources to compensate the birds' owners. All we know is that in autumn 2004, the disease returned to the villages around the Red River delta. Dr Pham Van Diu was appalled: 'The people here in Thai Binh are living in fear,' he said. 'They don't understand the virus. It's a mystery.'

THE NEW YEAR CELEBRATION, FEBRUARY 2005

Thirteen months after Ngo Le Hung's death, another young man in the same region found himself shivering, despite the heat. Twenty-one-year-old Nguyen Sy Tuan had been working on the coast, harvesting seaweed, but he returned home for the culmination of the traditional Lunar New Year celebrations on Tet, which in 2005 fell on 9 February. Nguyen Sy Tuan helped his mother to slaughter a duck, which he had bought from a neighbour. They poured its blood into a bowl and prepared a rich broth from it, a soup which is traditionally eaten the evening before Tet, and which has immense religious and traditional significance. The young man had the soup, and five days later he found himself unable to move from his bed.

He was admitted to Hanoi's Bach Mai Hospital where he became a patient of Dr Nguyen Thong Van, head of the hospital's intensive care unit and a remarkable woman who led the country's battle against the SARS epidemic in 2003. She didn't think Sy Tuan would survive, because the virus had spread quickly through his organs and, most dangerously, had infected his lungs. X-rays showed a white smudge covering both of his lungs. One of the big problems with bird flu is that the virus invites the body to trigger a huge defensive chemical reaction, so that the lungs are flooded with white blood cells which then cause a major inflammatory reaction. This kills healthy tissue and the blood vessels start to leak. The lungs fill with fluid and other agents, such as pneumococcal infections, can take advantage of the damage.

But, Dr Thong recalls: 'When it seemed the situation couldn't get much worse, it started to get better. Two weeks later, when he hadn't died, I thought maybe we could cure him.'

Sy Tuan's fourteen-year-old sister also contracted the virus.

Worryingly, she had had no contact with live or slaughtered birds. Her temperature soared to 105 degrees F, but the fever lasted for just four days. Like Tuan, she survived and when she returned to school, her friends had given her a new nickname – 'Miss H5' – after the H5N1 virus she had fought off.

The story of Sy Tuan and his sister should be a cause for celebration, but there is a darker side. A nurse at the hospital, who had been caring for Sy Tuan, became infected with the virus but survived after spending 82 days in hospital. *Guardian* journalists Adrian Levy and Cathy Scott-Clark tracked down the nurse in October 2005. He told them: 'I live in the hospital dorm and couldn't have come into contact with poultry, only nurses and patients.' He was asked to look after Sy Tuan for seven hours before he was isolated from the other patients. At the time, the nurse's case was never linked to the family, but it may be an ominous warning sign that the virus had finally found a way of leaping from person to person rather than just bird to person. However, this was never conclusively proven.

> *'At the time, the nurse's case was never linked to the family, but it may be an ominous warning sign that the virus had finally found a way of leaping from person to person rather than just bird to person.'*

MEDICAL FACILITIES IN VIETNAM

In North Vietnam, if flu patients are caught early enough, they often end up in the main intensive care unit of Hanoi's Bach Mai Hospital, where their chances of survival are highest. The first symptoms are usually a head cold, high fever and sneezing. Within one or two days, the patients suddenly find it difficult to breathe and their lungs begin to fail. Dr Nguyen Thong Van realized early on that the only hope for survival was to put the patients on ventilators as quickly as possible. 'We've treated seventeen cases,' she said, following an outbreak in early 2005. 'Three of them died because they suffered severe damage to other organs from the virus and then had a general collapse, rather like toxic shock.' But the rest survived, generally after a long period of hospitalization.

The West must invest

Dr Jeremy Farrar is director of Oxford University's Clinical Research Unit in Ho Chi Minh City, which is based at the city's Tropical Diseases Hospital. Dr Farrar believes the world could have done more to help the country:

'Money has to come from the West, from the EU or America, because we need investment to make it possible to diagnose illness more quickly, and then to offer the right critical care. Perhaps people don't realize it, but there are only three laboratories [in Vietnam] which can do any diagnostic testing.... But we are lucky, because in Cambodia there is only one laboratory. In Laos, I don't think there is even one.'

Dr Farrar believes that Western governments don't understand quite how hard it is to make the initial diagnosis, in a country where most people don't have easy access to a doctor or a health centre. 'It's a horrible infection as it develops, but in the early phase, when you are most infectious, it is just a fever and a cough. Millions of people in Asia live with that every day of the week. Also, you have to remember that there is no rapid diagnostic test available. So sometimes we hear of outbreaks in remote villages, and it is hard to respond, because it might be the rainy season, and the roads might be flooded, or you can't get through for some reason.'

As the country only has eight dollars to spend on the health of each citizen annually, it's not hard to see how the lack of resources has hindered their ability to deal with the disease.

In early 2005, at the Hospital for Tropical Diseases in Ho Chi Minh City, southern Vietnam, beds that were normally reserved for malaria patients were turned into a specialist isolation unit. Patients were given oxygen masks and ventilators. Nurses were given masks and gowns to protect themselves from the virus. All the same, nine patients were to die there over the next few months, one of them a girl of just eighteen years old; x-rays showed graphically how her lung tissue was destroyed over just four days. She was treated with oseltamivir (Tamiflu), an expensive anti-viral drug (see page 87), and put on a ventilator but it still wasn't enough to save her.

Although the Vietnamese government claimed in the autumn of 2005 to have the disease under control – they said the death rate had fallen to 20 per cent of infected cases – hospital staff still tell the same story, of patients coming in with flu symptoms but quickly deteriorating. At the time of writing, Vietnam has suffered more than 40 fatalities and they claim that all of the victims were apparently infected by chickens, but there is a suspicion that in at least two clusters it may have passed between humans. The case is not proven either because the WHO was not able to investigate, or the bodies of the victims had been cremated before they could be tested.

'There is also a suggestion that the virus in northern Vietnam is slightly different, slightly less virulent, than that in the south.'

Another aspect of the virus that puzzles the doctors is why some people appear to have immunity to it. One eleven-year-old Vietnamese girl survived against all the odds, and others have been found to have the antigens in their blood but are asymptomatic. Is it possible that some people in this region have built up an immunity to it, or are there genetic factors at play? There is also a suggestion that the virus in northern Vietnam is slightly different, slightly less virulent, than that in the south.

THE GREAT CULL, SEPTEMBER 2005

There was no relief for the many thousands of Vietnamese who live around the rice paddies and are dependent on poultry for their survival. In September 2005, officials finally began to get to grips with the enormous task of slaughtering millions of birds in affected areas and innoculating as many of their domestic poultry as possible with a vaccine to try and prevent the spread. Anton Rychener, the director of the UN Food and Agricultural Organization in Vietnam, who has constantly been telling the West that the solutions to tackling bird flu are not that simple, commented: 'It's a logistical nightmare. It's very, very difficult.

It's complex and it requires quite a bit of determination and funds.' There was barely a family left untouched by the huge initiative, in which 46 million ducks and chickens were killed, at a cost of $190 million, and 60 million birds were immunized.

In villages around the country, women and children could be seen clutching squealing chickens, or putting them in baskets on the backs of bicycles as they went off to receive the vaccine, administered by rural health workers in masks and gowns. For many families, the slaughter of ducks and chickens found to be infected had enormous economic consequences. It not only changed the farming practices and the lifestyle of their villages, but it also ravaged entire communities. Farmers who were surviving on a very basic wage were ordered to build pens to separate their poultry from human habitation instead of allowing them to roam freely in the backyards. The only place where duck eggs can be incubated now is in the large-scale breeding farms where vets can come in to test for the disease.

A high price to pay

For individuals, the cost is high. Nguyen Thi Hanh used to watch her flocks of ducks waddle across the road outside her house, in the tranquil village of Uong Bi in Quang Ninh province. But an outbreak of the disease in early 2005 meant that all her ducks and chickens had to be slaughtered. The slaughter cost them 20 million dong (around $1000), half the family's assets, and they were only paid the basic government compensation rate, which was between a quarter and a half of the birds' market value. The crisis caused the break-up of the family, as Hanh told Jonathan Watts, a Guardian journalist: 'Apart from a dozen birds in the yard, we've given up raising chickens. My husband has become a driver and my parents have moved south to look for work.'

There may be one more side effect of the great cull of poultry in rural Vietnam. One of the reasons why malnutrition rates had fallen so sharply across the region in recent decades was because of the wide availability of chicken, providing a fresh, plentiful source of eggs and nutritious meat. For most families, this was their main source of protein – the food that would help their children thrive and avoid many of the childhood diseases that are still endemic in the region. Living in a Western society with access to supermarkets selling an endless variety of food, it's very easy to forget that this is a luxury not shared by most of the world. Without their ducks and chickens, there could well be a return to higher rates of malnutrition in the poorest areas of Southeast Asia.

H5N1 IN THAILAND

Thailand, which neighbours Vietnam, claimed to have eradicated H5N1 from its poultry, but it is now clear that the disease was present in some poultry farms back in 2003. These cases were not reported to outside agencies such as the WHO or the World Organization for Animal Health (also known as OIE) and it seems that there was a cover-up as the authorities struggled to protect Thailand's lucrative poultry industry and its burgeoning number of 'super-farms' which process thousands of chickens a day for a global market. When chickens began to drop down dead on farms, it was initially claimed they were suffering from 'chicken cholera'. As the American author Mike Davis points out in his book *The Monster at Our Door* (The New Press, 2005), 'Lies were being manufactured almost as fast as sick chickens were being slaughtered and shipped to overseas markets.'

'Without their ducks and chickens, there could well be a return to higher rates of malnutrition in the poorest areas of Southeast Asia.'

The Thai Prime Minister went on national TV and ate a huge plate of Thai chicken to assuage a nervous public, in much the same way that back in 1990, the British agriculture minister John Selwyn Gummer was pictured by the *Sun* newspaper feeding a burger to his daughter Cordelia at the height of the BSE crisis, to 'prove' that beef was safe to eat. Both men were seriously misguided.

Early in 2004, two young farmers' sons died of bird flu and the Thai government was forced to admit there was a problem.

THE SPREAD AMONG BIRDS

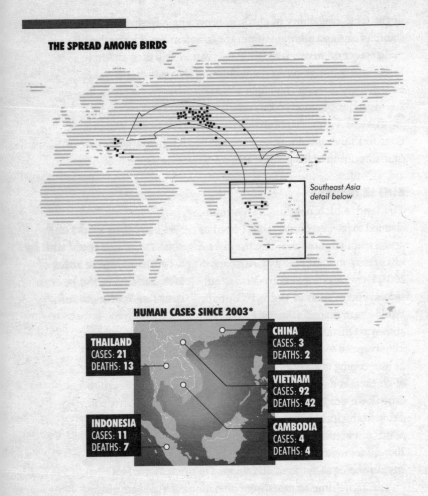

Southeast Asia
detail below

HUMAN CASES SINCE 2003*

CHINA
CASES: 3
DEATHS: 2

THAILAND
CASES: 21
DEATHS: 13

VIETNAM
CASES: 92
DEATHS: 42

INDONESIA
CASES: 11
DEATHS: 7

CAMBODIA
CASES: 4
DEATHS: 4

*Reported to the World Health Organization
as of 23 November 2005

The spread of bird flu   A map showing the spread of flu among birds and humans

Imports of Thai poultry were immediately banned in many countries, including the whole of the European Union. The Thai authorities took rapid steps to set up a massive surveillance programme
of its poultry flocks and cull any affected ones, a process they were
able to do more easily than their Vietnamese neighbours because
they are a much wealthier country.

Thousands of villagers were recruited to become chicken 'vig-
ilantes' and watch out for any unusual patterns of ill health. A
heavily publicized 'X-ray' programme was instigated and highly
trained officials were sent into all the villages to collect samples
from each flock. If ducks were found to harbour the disease, the entire
flock had to be culled, but farmers were fairly compensated. This
meant that the infection rate in ducks fell from nearly 40 per cent
in October 2004 to what is now said to be virtually undetectable levels. By throwing both money and resources at the problem, you can
virtually wipe it out in your domestic bird stocks. This probably
accounts for the fact that, to date, Thailand has only had twenty human
cases of bird flu and thirteen deaths, about a third of the number
of its neighbour, Vietnam. But many experts think it's likely that they
could have prevented the human deaths if they had acted sooner.

HOW BIRD FLU SPREAD ACROSS ASIA

Dr Robert Webster, avian influenza expert with St Jude Children's
Research Hospital in Memphis, Tennessee, commented: 'Flu, like
SARS, knows no borders, and it is likely that H5N1 will continue
to cross them. Consequently, relying on culling alone is a risky strategy.' In July 2004 he reported to colleagues that H5N1 had been
circulating in China from 2001 onwards, and that its pattern of timing and distribution 'coincides with the general period of winter
bird migration to southern China'.

The smuggling of birds across borders may be just as responsible as natural migration patterns. Vietnam shares more than
1000 km of border with China, and it is estimated that tonnes of
chickens were being smuggled across regularly in 2004, because it
was impossible to police every single shipment. There were accusations

in July of that year that Chinese smugglers had been selling diseased birds in the markets of the northern province of Bac Giang in Vietnam. If this is the case, the fault lies not only with those who police the borders but also with those in charge of inspecting the markets in question.

From the summer of 2004, several other countries began to report that they had been affected.

- In August 2004, a pair of Malaysian fighting cocks was found by vets to have the disease. They had just returned from a match in Thailand.

- The first cases in Cambodia didn't appear until December 2004 but at the time of writing, four humans have died of the disease there, all of them young – their ages ranged from eight to 28.

- North Korea, a notoriously secretive country, found an outbreak in March 2005 in Pyonyang, near its border with China, and slaughtered 219,900 chickens at three farms.

- Laos and Indonesia have both reported cases during 2005.

By the summer of 2005, the nature of the threat had become clearer to everyone. As the World Health Organization warned very bluntly in its document 'Responding to the avian influenza pandemic: recommended strategic actions', the risk is there for as long as the H5N1 virus continues to circulate in animals.

'Hopes that the virus could be rapidly eliminated from poultry have not been realized, and the situation has grown increasingly worrisome,' the document stated. 'The virus, in its highly pathogenic form, is now endemic in many parts of Indonesia and Vietnam and in some parts of Cambodia, China, Thailand and possibly also the Lao People's Democratic Republic. Factors responsible for persistence of the virus are not fully understood. The dynamics of H5N1 behaviour in animals are likewise poorly understood and unpredictable.'

It pointed out that waterfowl were emerging as a particular

risk factor. 'The fact that domestic ducks can act as a "silent" reservoir means there's no clear warning signal and there's more chance of unwitting human exposure, especially for rural farmers and their families.' Equally worrying is that other mammal species not thought to be susceptible have recently developed the disease. For example, some tigers in a Thai zoo have caught it, and studies in domestic cats show that they too can be infected.

As the report points out, there is a political reason why these outbreaks are sometimes kept 'silent'. The persistence of the virus has put some nations under severe economic strain. 'An inability adequately to compensate farmers for lost birds reduces the incentive to report outbreaks, particularly in rural areas where the true risk of human exposure resides.'

What is now becoming clear is that during the six-year 'silence' between the first outbreak in Hong Kong and its re-emergence in the rice paddies of Vietnam, the disease was not sleeping at all. It was busy infecting wild birds in China, Cambodia and Thailand and it was also appearing in the many millions of birds kept as domestic poultry across the region.

'An inability adequately to compensate farmers for lost birds reduces the incentive to report outbreaks, particularly in rural areas where the true risk of human exposure resides.'

CHINA: THE GREAT UNKNOWN

China, a nation where there are vast contrasts between the modern cities and the poor rural areas, is still a closed society. Its astonishing rise as a superpower and the creation of ever-expanding cities founded on the electronics and textiles industries, has led to an enormous migration of people out of the farms and into the factories.

But even though its wealth has grown massively, China's ability to monitor the emergence of new diseases is still very poor. Many millions of inhabitants have no health insurance and cannot afford to see a doctor. So far, there have been no recorded, official cases of bird flu affecting Chinese people, although there have been rumours circulating for more than a year that there have been cases.

Back in May 2005, hundreds of wild geese were found dead on

the shores of the Qinghai Lake Nature Reserve (see page 71). A second outbreak of bird flu occurred in Tacheng City, near the border with Kazakhstan, more than 1600 km east of the lake. Chinese authorities attempted to dampen down fears by claiming that the outbreak was under control, and that no humans had been affected or were in danger. Meanwhile, the Beijing government approved a sales permit for a new vaccine which would halt the spread of the virus in birds (it doesn't work on people). No one knows how effective this vaccine is because it hasn't been evaluated outside China, but supplies of the vaccine have been sent to farms around the affected regions. The plan was to vaccinate 3 million birds, and particularly to stop the disease spreading from migratory birds, such as geese, to the resident waterfowl, which could easily pass it on to domestic flocks. The problem with vaccination, however, is that a bird can carry the virus without showing any symptoms. The disease is thus disguised, rather than eradicated.

'The problem with vaccination, however, is that a bird can still carry the virus even though they won't show any symptoms. The disease is thus disguised, rather than eradicated.'

International concern about the way in which China deals with health threats is high, not least because of its handling of the SARS epidemic in 2003. Officials and politicians covered up the epidemic when it emerged in southern regions of China, and failed to tell international authorities what was happening. The health minister was eventually dismissed as China faced worldwide condemnation for its secretive attitude, and the Beijing government promised to be more open about such problems in the future.

But history shows that the country remains less than helpful in its dealings with international bodies. In May 2005, the UN's Food and Agriculture Organization was not informed of an enormous cull of cattle following a serious outbreak of foot-and-mouth disease in northern China. With bird flu, very few outside experts have been allowed in to investigate how endemic the virus is within domestic poultry flocks.

The opportunities for the virus to spread from wild to domestic birds and back again is simply greater in China than anywhere else in the world. It has a population of 1.3 billion and raises around ten times that number of poultry, most of them on small farms. For centuries, the hens have been kept in the yard or in pens next to ducks and pigs, but recently poultry-rearing has become a major industry, with huge commercial farms providing cheaper meat, without necessarily complying with the hygiene standards that would be compulsory in a European country. As the country's economy grows at such a rapid rate, so do the demands for cheap and protein-rich meat, no matter how it is supplied.

China's responsibility to the world

Professor David Ho, influenza expert and scientific director of the Aaron Diamond AIDS Research Centre at Rockefeller University in New York, warned back in May 2005 in a commentary for the journal Nature that China has to improve its ability to spot emerging diseases. 'China's recent SARS-fighting experience will give its pandemic response an edge. But this advantage will be offset by a number of factors: China is likely to be hit first or early by the pandemic; its disease-surveillance system and overall healthcare infrastructure are inadequate; the health authorities have yet to come up with a detailed strategic preparedness plan; and it has limited technical resources to produce enough vaccines and drugs to combat the pandemic.' He added, ominously: 'There is little doubt that China will be in deep trouble if the flu pandemic were to strike in the next few years. It has a moral obligation to its own people, and to the world, to rectify the situation as soon as possible.'

There are some encouraging signs. In October 2005, Chinese official Hui Liangyu admitted that China now faces a 'grave' threat from bird flu. He said his country was intensifying its battle against the virus, by introducing more rigorous monitoring and immunization of birds. 'We cannot let down our guard, we cannot underestimate the risks of the outbreaks,' he said.

Then in November 2005, the health ministry reported that a 24-year-old female poultry worker in the eastern province of Anhui, had died after being infected with the H5N1 strain of bird flu. A nine-year-old boy called He Junyao had also contracted the virus in a different region, the Hunan province, but recovered despite contracting pneumonia. His sister, He Yin, however, fell ill and died. It is suspected she too had bird flu, but her body was cremated before samples could be taken. The boy and the woman were the first two reported cases of human bird flu in China.

EUROPE'S WORST NIGHTMARE

The tiny Greek island of Inousses is about as close to a Mediterranean paradise as you can find. This tranquil spot, near the coast of Turkey, is known for its clear waters and sheltered shores. Down the generations it has provided Greece with many of her wealthiest shipping families, and several streets are named after the renowned Pateras clan. But now it is famous for another reason. A small farm there became the first place in the European Union to harbour the lethal strain of H5N1.

In October 2005, Dimitris Komninaris found that his turkeys were sick, and some had died. He told local vets, who immediately sent off samples and found what everyone had been dreading, that one of the turkeys that died was carrying H5 antibodies. A team of experts clad in protective boiler-suits was sent in to disinfect the farm.

Despite the fact that the turkeys were not even part of an export business – all were used for the family's own consumption – the local prefect Polidoras Lambrinoudis instituted an immediate ban on any poultry or eggs leaving the tiny island, which has only 500 inhabitants. But the effect of this single infection was to be far, far wider. Bulgaria banned the imports of all live fowl, poultry products and eggs from Greece as well as prohibiting the transit of any lorries carrying birds that had passed through Turkey, Greece or Romania. And as the residents of Inousses were reeling from the shock of visits from vets, doctors and even the government health minister, more bad news broke out. In Kiziksa in western Turkey, bird flu was discovered on a turkey farm (see page 72). A week later it was reported that a number of birds had died in the city of Bitola, Macedonia, near the border with Greece, and samples were being sent to a British laboratory in Weybridge for further testing.

Since September 2004, the disease had been hitchhiking its way westwards across continents, with each new rumour of an outbreak sparking fears, as well as tough farming restrictions to protect national economies. It is always the smallholders and local communities who are worst affected. To see your entire flock being destroyed because of a contagion which until yesterday seemed a distant threat is an acutely painful and sad event. Watching men in green plastic suits and masks going into your home to disinfect it with special sprays must be terrifying. For some, it must seem like the end of a way of life.

> '*Since September 2004, the disease had been hitchhiking its way westwards across continents, with each new rumour of an outbreak sparking fears, as well as tough farming restrictions to protect national economies.*'

Romania found out it had birds infected with H5N1 back in October 2005, along the beautiful green waters of the Danube delta. Thousands of birds land there every autumn, before travelling inland to feed on the maize and barley crops. This has become yet another area blighted by avian flu, although it hasn't infected a single human being. Anyone leaving or entering the area now has to walk through pools of disinfectant. Every car and lorry – even the trains – are sprayed with chemicals. The Romanians are taking no chances. They have had to cull thousands of birds – and if another outbreak is found, will have to cull thousands more.

Lefter Chirica, the government-appointed official responsible for Romania's Tulcea district, surveyed the police and border guards patrolling the villages of Maliuc and Vulturu. 'I never thought it would come to this,' he told BBC News. 'It's like a science fiction film – men in strange overalls, walking through our villages.'

Creating barriers between wild and domestic birds is an almost impossible task in an area such as the Danube, or the Red River delta of Vietnam, or in the wetlands of Cambodia. Each country has done its best, but will it be enough to prevent the virus from mutating further and becoming a fully human pathogen? In Chapter 6, I will explain how other nations, so far free of the disease, have attempted to prevent the mixing of different bird species, with some taking drastic measures and others doing very little at all. Each time the story moves to a different nation, more heartache is seen – and the world is nudged slightly closer to the chances of a human flu pandemic.

4 HOW WILD GEESE BROUGHT THE VIRUS TO OUR DOORSTEP

'This virus has been around for eight years and so far hasn't proved to be lethally transmissible from birds to people. But of course, we don't know how long the evolution of a pandemic strain takes, do we? We weren't able to study the last one in such detail.'

Dr Ian Brown   Head of Avian Virology, Veterinary Laboratory Agency, UK

There are few places in the world more beautiful than the Qinghai Lake nature reserve in northwest China. Thousands of foreign tourists head to this desolate spot every year, in order to enjoy the wonderful spectacle of birds gliding over the immense stretch of salt water. It is a birdwatchers' paradise, which more than 200 species use to hatch their young after their long flights across Asia.

But back in May 2005, one of the wardens noticed something strange. A bar-headed goose was walking in an unusual manner, swaying from side to side. It looked to Li Yinghua, the ranger who saw him, almost as if the bird was shivering. It was taken in to be cared for, but died soon afterwards. Over the next six weeks, thousands of other birds around the lake suffered the same fate. Some mysterious illness was spreading among them, as they shared their nesting grounds and their food. Most of the affected birds were bar-headed geese, a breed of waterfowl that is particularly elegant but seems susceptible to new infections.

It was not until the end of June that the Chinese authorities allowed the World Health Organization onto the reserve to investigate the situation. When they did, the enormity of the problem became apparent. The samples taken from all of the dead birds showed that the highly pathogenic form of H5N1 had infected them.

THE VIRUS TRAVELS WEST

The H5N1 subtype of bird flu has now spread at a fairly alarming rate through nine different Asian countries. Perhaps it hitchhikes a ride with wild birds as they wing their way over national borders, or perhaps there are other more secret routes of transmission – the illegal smuggling of live birds, for example – that have escalated the spread. We may never know exactly how this chain of infection worked, but we do know that between 1997 and 2005 it was found in bird populations in Mongolia, Siberia, Tibet and Kazakhstan. By the autumn of 2005, it had reached Europe's doorstep, with domestic poultry becoming infected in Romania, Turkey, Greece and, most recently, Croatia.

The poor villagers of Kiziksa in western Turkey had no idea what was happening to them. It seemed like the act of a vengeful god. One unlucky farmer, Mehmet Eksen, told the BBC in October 2005 that he knew something was wrong when 50 of his turkeys fell ill and died in the space of a day. Another hundred died the next day. 'I thought they'd been poisoned, so I treated them with ayran [a yoghurt drink] at first,' he explained.

This didn't work, so he reported the deaths to local vets, who immediately suspected the worst and instituted a cull of thousands of birds in the region. All poultry had to be taken to the town square for slaughter and those farmers who failed to comply with the regulations faced six months in jail. Among the villagers there was widepread suspicion about the tests and their results. 'Why did no other birds die?' demanded one man angrily. 'Our healthy chickens are being slaughtered for nothing.'

Kiziksa is close to a national park called, ironically enough, Bird Paradise. It is on a flightpath commonly used by many species of geese as they prepare for the winter months and it is strongly suspected that wild birds flying south from Russia for the winter caused the contagion there.

There has long been concern about the possibility of migratory birds carrying the disease, although until recently very little had been done about it. In 2004 a scientific paper published by Dr Robert Webster of St Jude Children's Research Hospital in Memphis, Tennessee warned that his research indicated that some birds could act as 'Trojan ducks'. They could harbour the virus without showing any symptoms. Until then, experts had believed that infected birds would drop dead fairly quickly, and therefore wouldn't be able to fly very far. Dr Webster's findings were alarming in the extreme.

THE VIRUS-HUNTER

Albert Osterhaus, the man who helped to identify H5N1 in Hong Kong in 1997, has long been worried about the possibility of wild birds spreading the infection. A veterinarian by training who switched to virology, he has spent his career tracking down animal viruses, watching them shift shape and lethality as they move between species and between countries. More than anyone else, he has tried to warn politicians – and his fellow animal and human health experts – that bird flu has a way of breaking all the normal rules.

'We know that viruses that start off as fairly harmless in birds can "heat up" when they reach poultry,' he explained. 'It's a real threat now. We need to be thinking about how we collect the data on outbreaks in poultry, and we need experts in the fields of human and animal health to work together far more closely than they have in the past.'

Dozens of different subtypes of flu exist in the guts of wild birds, and can be harmless to them. But occasionally there will be one that crosses over into domestic birds, where it can do far more damage. Wild bird droppings, either on land or in the water, can harbour particles of the virus for two days. When a wild bird lands close to a domesticated hen, the hen can become infected through contact with the droppings, or through shed feathers, or even by the air exhaled by the wild bird.

In early 2003, Dr Osterhaus and his team at the Erasmus Medical Center in Rotterdam got a foretaste of exactly how serious it can be when bird flu strikes. On 28 February, he took a call from a colleague at the Dutch Ministry of Agriculture telling him that they had heard about a farm where the chickens were dying of something odd. 'They were going to wait over the weekend before sending me the samples on Monday and I said, "No, don't wait, send me all five chickens today."'

'When a wild bird lands close to a domesticated hen, the hen can become infected through contact with the droppings, or through shed feathers, or even by the air exhaled by the wild bird.'

His speedy laboratory work over that weekend confirmed that the chickens were infected with the subtype H7N7, a potentially lethal form of bird flu. Osterhaus had to persuade the health authorities to take it seriously and issued orders that all workers, especially those culling the infected birds, should wear protective clothing, gloves and masks before they went onto the farms.

Some colleagues thought he was over-reacting but his arguments convinced them, and the farm workers who had been exposed to the chickens were given anti-viral drugs as a preventive measure. That bird flu virus ended up infecting 89 people, but because of the very rapid practical precautions they took only one 57-year-old man died.

'We started work on February 28, and by March 1 we had our first clinical case, a worker with conjunctivitis,' recalled Osterhaus. 'We also had just one fatal case but it was very sad. A vet who had been at a farm where the infection had not yet been confirmed developed pneumonia. His lungs were loaded with the virus, which was eating away at the pneumocytes [lung cells]. The lungs started leaking and basically when that happens, you drown in the fluid.'

At the Erasmus Medical Center they have 30,000 samples of duck tissue, painstakingly collected by ornithologists and others, which they analyze by purifying it, collecting the genetic material and then identifying any viruses. So far, the number of samples collected that have tested positive for some kind of influenza virus runs at between 2 and 20 per cent, depending on the species of bird.

Dr Osterhaus thinks it is only a matter of time before the pandemic comes. 'Flu is knocking on the door,' he said bluntly. In a commentary in the journal *Nature* in May 2005, he called for the institution of an international task force which could be sent in to investigate outbreaks. Both veterinarians and doctors could then brief local authorities on the best ways of collecting data, monitoring further outbreaks, and carrying out post-mortems on those who die from the disease. His pleas for such a task force have so far fallen on deaf ears, but surely the story of how Dr Osterhaus's team fought H7N7 in 2003 should alert officials everywhere to the need for immediate action as soon as symptoms are seen in just one bird, because any delay at all can prove fatal.

> **'Dr Osterhaus thinks it is only a matter of time before the pandemic comes. "Flu is knocking on the door," he said bluntly.'**

THE FLIGHTPATHS TAKEN BY GEESE

Every year, millions of birds fly on different routes around the world to nest and breed. There are many thousands of flightpaths running north to south and east to west, but still relatively little is known about how many birds follow each route, or how and why they diverge to other areas. Our knowledge of migration comes mainly from birdwatchers and ornithologists who compare notes and report their findings. Some have systems of migration surveillance that involve placing rings on birds' legs, so that when they have flown elsewhere and the rings are monitored by authorities at their stopping places, information can be recorded about the route they have taken. But the amount of ringing each year is minuscule compared with the actual numbers flying.

One of the biggest worries at the moment is that the virus

could be winging its way to Africa, a continent which is almost completely unprepared to deal with the threat of a lethal strain of flu. Wild birds could easily spread it by leaving droppings in or near the large lakes that are shared by waterfowl and domestic poultry. Joseph Domenech, the chief veterinary officer for the UN's Food and Agriculture Organisation (FAO) has expressed his concerns about what might happen next. 'Wild birds seem to be one of the main avian influenza carriers, but more research is urgently needed to fully understand their role in spreading the virus... One of our major concerns is now the potential spread of avian influenza through migratory birds to northern and eastern Africa. There is a serious risk that this scenario may become a reality.' He wants to see the Middle East and northern Africa building up a line of defence against the virus, supported by other countries, so that their vets can be on the look-out for the first signs in both wild and domestic birds.

'The virus could be winging its way to Africa, a continent which is almost completely unprepared to deal with the threat of a lethal strain of flu.'

Many birds migrating from Asia to the northern hemisphere stop off in the freshwater ponds, dams and lakes along East Africa's Rift Valley. This spectacular geographical feature runs for 5000 km from north to south, all the way from Syria into Mozambique. The burden of AIDS and malaria in rural populations in the Valley is already very high and the concept of bio-security on farms has barely been heard of, so an outbreak of avian flu could be utterly devastating.

'We have been discussing the issue almost every night. We pray it doesn't come here,' said Aka Sekalala, managing director of Ugachick, Uganda's biggest poultry breeder. 'At least in Europe they can pay people something for the birds if they have to be destroyed, but here we would just collapse,' he told Reuters. 'It would be terrible.'

Jacques Diouf, director-general of the FAO, has expressed his frustration at the focus on human health and the lack of support for veterinarians. In October 2005 he announced that, together with the World Organization for Animal Health, they have developed a detailed global strategy for the control of avian influenza in animals and have calculated the cost of implementation at about $175 million (US) to support surveillance, diagnosis and other control measures such as vaccination. 'We are still facing a serious funding gap and have only received around $30 million to date from Germany, Japan, the Netherlands, Switzerland and the United States,' he explained. 'We can't afford to wait to battle the disease in pharmacies and hospitals; we need to get rid of the virus in affected farmers' backyards. In the end, prevention will be cheaper than the cure.'

WHAT CAN FARMERS DO NOW?

For farmers around the world, the possibility that a highly pathogenic form of H5N1 might infect domestic poultry flocks is one that they can hardly bear to contemplate. As the disease has moved to Europe, agricultural organizations across the EU have been putting up defences. In some cases, they have done so literally.

In the wake of the Netherlands outbreak of H7N7 back in 2003, drastic action was taken. All farms there were instructed to build completely indoor facilities, which must also accommodate the country's 5 million-plus free-range hens. Bio-security is of the utmost importance in a country where there are 100 million hens and just 16 million human beings. Some parts of Germany have followed suit – one province has built hundreds of indoor facilities for its birds – and in October 2005, 21 different *départements* in France did the same, ordering farmers and breeders to keep their birds indoors.

In Britain, the Department for the Environment, Food and Rural Affairs (Defra), has so far held back from ordering all poultry flocks indoors as a precautionary measure. As one Whitehall insider put it to me: 'We are damned if we do, and damned if we don't. If we do this too soon, it will look like a panic measure and could cause enormous economic harm. If we don't, and it comes here, it might mean an awful lot of culling.'

In October 2005, the British government advised: 'Anyone who

The British flu detective

Deep in the Surrey countryside, Dr Ian Brown and a team of 24 staff at the Veterinary Laboratory Agency (VLA) in Weybridge are at the forefront of attempts to diagnose suspected cases of bird flu as quickly and accurately as possible. Theirs is the central avian flu reference laboratory for the whole of Europe, and they often give up their weekends in order to analyse the samples from dead birds sent to them from around the world as quickly as possible.

For Dr Brown, a modest but cheerful man who is also a keen birdwatcher, it seems as if his whole career has led him to this point. 'It's very challenging and very rewarding. Once you get working on influenza, you don't move into anything else,' he told me. 'We don't do this for the financial incentives – you do it because you really want to feel you can make a difference.'

Working in a sealed room so that none of the microbes can escape to the outside world, in conditions below atmospheric pressure, his team examines samples of tissue and faeces taken from diseased birds, sequences the genes and works out the level of threat each represents. The diagnosis they make will have profound consequences for many countries, both economic and psychological.

Although it has only relatively recently become known around the world, bird flu is nothing new to Dr Brown. Since the early 1970s he has been studying its different varieties, and looking at their effects inside the gut of a chicken. 'Our perception is that this [H5N1] is a virus which has been around in poultry for a long time, maybe not the subtype which is in Asia right now, but of the same serotype.' He describes the 1997 Hong Kong outbreak as a 'really significant event' because until then, no one had imagined it could leap the species barrier in such a way. After that things seemed to go quiet, until it re-emerged in late 2003 in Thailand and in early 2004 in Vietnam. 'It's difficult to be really accurate about what was happening in those years, because you are relying on the transparency and the reports coming out of these countries. But they don't necessarily have that transparency.'

I asked him what was happening in China. Was the disease endemic there in their chicken flocks? He replied: 'We are unclear what kind of surveillance work is going on there. I am aware that they are doing some, but are they going into the markets, and taking samples? We don't know. The problem for the WHO is that they don't have a good picture of what is going on in China either. Certainly three or four years ago, China didn't see influenza as a big problem.'

From 1997 onwards, there has been a plethora of new variants of H5N1, caused when the droppings of wild birds are ingested or inhaled by poultry which can then act as the mixing vessels for a new form to emerge. Although it is easy to blame migratory waterfowl, they are not the only culprits. What is becoming increasingly clear is that globally, there are thousands of shipments of live birds each year, which often go unchecked for disease.

Despite its international reputation, Dr Brown's team did not receive its first sample of H5N1 material until March 2004. 'To be honest, we only got that because the European Union dug its heels in with Thailand and said that under a trade agreement, the material had to be sent out and investigated,' said Dr Brown. 'I don't know how long it would have taken otherwise.'

Samples of infected poultry taking too long to reach labs, or not reaching labs at all, is a hot political issue. If there have been long delays before scientists were able to examine infected human tissue, then those delays are magnified many times when it comes to birds. Some countries, such as Cambodia, were suspicious of the motives lying behind attempts to check their birds. And, as Dr Brown points out, there is also the question of intellectual property rights. If a lab has a sample of the virus, it would be possible for an unscrupulous

(continued over)

researcher to manufacture a vaccine containing the antigenic properties needed to combat that particular strain and then demand the kind of money for it that many countries couldn't afford to pay.

H5N1 is changing itself all the time, and it is known that several varieties exist within birds. It isn't known which species carry the virus, or why it might be so varied. 'We know that the birds that were found at the Qinghai Lake [in China] had a different variation of the virus from others,' said Dr Brown. 'This suggests it had got into another population of birds and had moved forward. Greater diversity in the reservoir of wild birds could be a bad sign, but at the moment we just don't know whether that makes it more transmissible to humans.'

Unlike some other experts, Dr Brown does not believe that it is a foregone conclusion that bird flu will make the leap to become a fully pandemic strain of flu.

---

keeps chickens or turkeys should look out for the following symptoms: noisy breathing and difficulty in breathing; a darkening of combs and wattles; diarrhoea; a drop in yield of eggs; dullness and lack of appetite.'

Many individual farmers have started to take their own biosecurity measures, such as using netting to make sure that wild birds can't land near their flocks. Poultry are also being fed and watered inside to deter any wild birds from being tempted to share the feed. Even potholes and puddles which could attract migrant species for a bathe are being filled in.

The head of the National Farmers' Union Tim Bennett has been in talks with Tony Blair over the measures that need to be taken. Above all, farmers want to avoid bird flu becoming another national crisis. The foot and mouth outbreak of 2001 showed that diseased animals not only put people off eating meat, but also stopped hundreds of thousands of tourists from visiting the British countryside.

It is deeply ironic that in October 2005, just as bird flu stories were hitting the headlines, the major supermarkets revealed that sales of free-range eggs had overtaken the sales of eggs from caged birds for the first time. The demand for good animal welfare is high, but poultry farmers have now been warned that they may have to make emergency preparations to bring indoors millions of birds that are currently free to run around outside.

Some believe this is just a panic measure. As Robin Maynard of the Soil Association said: 'You have a situation where you are being told avian flu could reach here in a year, or five or ten. Do farmers have to keep their poultry inside all that time? If you do this you would be destroying the most successful part of the farming sector – the growth of free range and organic.'

But is it better to be safe than sorry?

'Anyone who keeps chickens or turkeys should look out for the following symptoms: noisy breathing and difficulty in breathing; a darkening of combs and wattles; diarrhoea; a drop in yield of eggs; dullness and lack of appetite.'

CHICKENS IN THE BACK YARD

No one knows exactly how many British people keep chickens in their gardens, but it is said to be the fastest-growing hobby in the UK. Estimates of numbers range from 200,000 to 500,000, and it is thought that only 6 per cent of poultry owners in the UK are actually known to Defra.

The message boards on some of the poultry-keeping websites are full of messages from concerned owners who are confused about what to do. On the Practical Poultry website, one man relates that the children's zoo at his work has been offered a family's pet ducks and hens because their neighbours are scared the birds will give them avian flu.

For many, their hens and roosters are family pets. Children learn how to look after them and collect the eggs and the whole family's emotional attachment to the birds is clear from some of

The poultry breeders

For some people, breeding poultry is much more than a hobby. Twenty years ago, Sue and Shaun Hammon gave up a busy life in London to head for the hills and raise chickens. They now run the Wernlas Collection, one of the top centres in Britain for conserving traditional and rare breeds of poultry.

They supply eggs or chickens to hundreds of poultry enthusiasts all over the country, from the person who wants a few hens in the back garden, to pub landlords who like to have decorative birds ranging around their gardens, as well as welcoming visitors who want to see the amazing plumage of the birds.

Their farm, nestling in the Shropshire Hills, presents an idyllic scene to visitors. There are more than 200 pens housing different species, from the Cuckoo Silkie and the Derbyshire Redcap to the Black-gold Araucana. All the birds have long runs, and can wander freely over the grass.

Sue Hammon is terrified by the prospect of bird flu coming into poultry in Britain. 'This is our livelihood and if they brought in new measures to order everyone to take their hens indoors, we couldn't do it. It would be absolutely impossible for us. For a start, we don't have the indoor facilities, but also the birds would fight if they were put together.' She believes that too much publicity has already been given to the disease. 'The media hype has been pretty grim. There is a lot of very frightening information coming out , and they are overplaying the situation. There was a different strain that affected Holland two years ago, and the disease didn't get any further.'

'It's a huge hobby now, keeping chickens,' Sue explains. 'Many of our customers say they want fresh eggs, because they are disenchanted with the supermarkets. But this scare is threatening all of that.' Certainly, for the Hammons it seems as though their whole way of life could be under threat.

the messages on websites, such as the BBC News site. Alex in Swansea wrote: 'I have 11 free range hens in a large enclosure open at the top to wild birds, who are in there stealing food every day. We live on the edge of a huge National Trust wetland habitat, with a large range of migratory species visiting throughout the year. I am extremely fond of these chickens, some of which we have raised from eggs, and my kids love them to bits. But if an order comes out from Defra, I will submit to the cull. Anything else would be wholly irresponsible.'

Johannes Paul of Omlet, a company that makes hi-tech chicken runs, says he advises customers to check the Defra website regularly and to be vigilant for signs of illness in their birds. 'It is extremely unlikely that an infected Canada goose will land in your garden. If it does spread here, the stereotypical British housewife will come into her own and barricade the hens to keep them safe,' he told BBC News.

THE TRADE IN EXOTIC BIRDS

In October 2005 Britain was shaken by the news that a parrot that died in quarantine in Essex was found to have the lethal form of H5N1. It raised enormous questions about the worldwide trade in exotic birds, a trade that has long been of concern to health experts.

However, it transpired that tissue samples between all the birds held in the quarantine centre at the same time had been mixed up, and it now seems it was some Mesia finches from Taiwan, rather than the Surinam parrot, that were the most likely source of the H5N1 virus. Environment Secretary Margaret Beckett ordered a review of quarantine procedures in Britain, amid concern about how such confusion could have arisen. The results of that review are due at the end of 2005.

The incident also led to a temporary ban on the import of all captive birds into the EU from around the world. As nearly 1 million birds and exotic pets are brought into the EU every year, this affects a sizeable number of creatures. There was also a ban on all bird fairs, exhibitions and shows, in order to prevent different birds from mixing and potentially spreading viruses in an enclosed space.

The Royal Society for the Protection of Birds (RSPB), one of Britain's biggest conservation organizations, believes it is imperative that the ban is made permanent.

Vigilance is the key

Mark Avery, director of conservation policy at the RSPB, said: 'The trade in wild birds is really quite crazy. The idea that you can take them from a jungle in South America, pack them up in a box in ghastly conditions where a number of them will die, and ship them round the world, so that they can sit in a cage in someone's front room for the rest of their life, is indefensible. It is also a means by which the virus could leapfrog the normal route and end up halfway round the world in no time.'

As a keen birdwatcher himself, Mark Avery believes that the key to ensuring that bird flu doesn't come to Britain is good surveillance. 'We have nature reserve wardens looking out for any suspicious deaths in birds, and if they find one, sending it off to be tested. Our general understanding of which species of birds migrate, and where and when they arrive here, is quite good. What we don't yet know is which species may be the most likely carriers of the virus.'

Among scientists, there is also concern that the focus has fallen on wild birds when it is still unclear how man-made problems may have helped the virus spread. William Karesh, director of the field veterinary programme of the Wildlife Conservation Society, said: 'We are wasting valuable time pointing fingers at wild birds when we should be focussing on dealing with the root causes of this epidemic spread which are clearly to be found in rural practices, the movement of domestic poultry and farming methods which crowd huge numbers of animals into small areas where they are more susceptible to disease.'

All in all, it appears likely that the battle against bird flu is going to have to be fought on more than one front.

A WILDLIFE SPECTACLE TURNED SOUR

Pochards, pintails, shovellers and tufted ducks: these are just some of the intriguingly named kinds of waterfowl that come to Britain every winter, winging their way across Europe to find the right grounds for the colder weather. Many of them end up in Slimbridge in Gloucestershire, at a bird reserve founded by the famous naturalist and ornithologist Sir Peter Scott. The son of Captain Scott of the Antarctic, this eminent man realized that birds needed a protected breeding ground on the banks of the Severn Estuary. The Wildfowl and Wetlands Trust (WWT) he set up here in 1946 has become the country's largest wildfowl sanctuary, with an important conservation role. It is a delight to walk around its 800 acres, and to watch the swans, geese and even the large gatherings of flamingoes who stop off here.

'In October 2005 Dr Ruth Cromie, waterbird research biology manager at WWT, started the unenviable task of co-ordinating efforts to catch 2000 of these birds and, as she delicately puts it, "wipe their bottoms".'

But it is here that the search for H5NI is beginning in the UK. In October 2005 Dr Ruth Cromie, waterbird research biology manager at WWT, started the unenviable task of co-ordinating efforts to catch 2000 of these birds and, as she delicately puts it, 'wipe their bottoms'. More scientifically, she was swabbing the birds in order to see if any faecal material contained particles of the virus. She feels perturbed by the way the virus has spread but still feels there is a low risk of it coming to the UK. 'You would expect to find some viruses there, because we all carry things around. Some of these birds will have low pathogenic strains – some H5, H1 or H2 kinds. But will it be the highly pathogenic form of H5N1? That's the million-dollar question.'

Dr Cromie, who has advised a government committee on the best ways to carry out surveillance work on migratory birds, thinks not. 'I feel the risk is low at the moment, but we have to be vigilant.'

Her most difficult task has been to devise ways of catching the birds without harming them. The traditional duck trap is a device into which they can be lured by means of food. There is a similar trap for swimming birds known as a swan pipe, which consists of a funnel-like contraption leading into a smaller cage. Then there is the alarming-sounding cannon-net. This is a means of catching the waterfowl while they are grazing on the ground. A net attached to a projectile is fired at speed so that it lands over the bird before it can fly off. After capture, the waterfowl – including mallards, widgeons and shovellers – are swabbed and ringed so that an accurate record can be made. If any of them are found to be carrying the lethal form of flu, it would be a very black day for the Wildfowl and Wetlands Trust.

'It is easy to blame the wild birds, and you can't do anything about it, but this disease has come from domestic poultry flocks,' commented Dr Cromie. 'It would be so sad if people started to associate negative ideas with the beautiful sight of these birds flying across the water.'

Everyone is hoping desperately that H5N1 won't have the devastating effects on wild bird species that some scientists are warning of – effects that could even mean some become extinct.

Species of waterbirds already under threat of extinction and now vulnerable to bird flu:

- *Dalmatian pelican*
- *Red-breasted goose*
- *Siberian crane*
- *Marbled teal*
- *White-headed duck*
- *Swinhoe's rail*
- *Sociable lapwing*
- *Spoon-billed sandpiper*

5 THE HUNT FOR A CURE

'Unlike the situation before previous flu pandemics, we now have the knowledge and technology to develop countermeasures for this deadly disease. However, unless we improve our capacity to produce such countermeasures, we may experience again the devastation of past pandemics.'

| Dr Anthony Fauci | Director of the National Institute of Allergy and Infectious Diseases, Maryland, US |

It would be hard for anyone not to have heard or read about the anti-viral drug Tamiflu in recent months. Also known as oseltamivir, it's the medication that currently provides one of the few defences the world has against a flu pandemic. Doctors have been able to prescribe it for the past three years to treat normal, seasonal flu in the elderly or patients at risk of complications, but the drug has also been shown to give some protection against bird flu, by reducing its severity. Governments are now racing to stockpile it as they come under pressure to have some form of medical protection in place.

Tamiflu is not a cure for bird flu, however. If we have a pandemic, it is not going to give anyone guaranteed protection. The drug relieves symptoms and cuts the complication rates for all kinds of influenza strains, but it has to be taken quickly – within two days of the first symptoms appearing – and even then it may only reduce by half the numbers needing hospital care. Amid all the hype over the drug, there remain huge uncertainties about how much such anti-viral medication will help us. The truth is that scientists simply do not know how big a weapon it is going to prove in our armoury against a pandemic. But any protection is better than nothing, and the entire globe wants it.

How much would you pay for a packet of ten tiny capsules that might end up saving your life in a flu pandemic? Back in 2004, you could have paid as little as $10 for them, because they were just another treatment that could reduce the severity of flu symptoms. Now, the price is anything between $70 and $200 a packet. The number of drug prescriptions written in America leapt by 710 per cent in the year to October 2005, as more and more people read about it. Roche, the company that makes it, watched its share price touch an all-time high last autumn as the world went crazy for the drug.

William Burns, head of pharmaceuticals at Roche said: 'Following four ducks in Romania carrying avian flu, Europe has gone mad. I don't think it is possible to find a single packet of Tamiflu in Paris any more.'

INSIDE THE ROCHE FACTORY

Star anise, a rare herb grown in China, has been valued down the centuries for the delicate, liquorice-like flavour it adds to meat dishes. This star-shaped plant, which is harvested between March and May each year, may look unremarkable, but its value now is incalculable because it is the only natural source of shikimic acid, from which the drug Tamiflu is made.

In a rather starkly designed factory on the outskirts of Basel, Switzerland, the capsules that everyone wants are being packaged up in tiny silver-foil strips. Each little blister pack contains ten capsules, which are half yellow and half light grey. Up and down a production line, you can watch the tiny lozenge-shaped drugs as they tumble through a vat and land in the middle of their own little indentation, which is then covered in tin foil, with the Roche logo stamped on the top. This is the last stage of production, which comes twelve months after the star anise has been picked off its branch.

With remarkable Swiss precision, nothing here is left to chance. There are thirteen factories involved in the production of oseltamivir, and they run 24 hours a day, seven days a week. By the end of 2006, they will be able to produce more than 300 million treatment courses of the drug each year.

In the lab, the shikimic acid is extracted from the star anise in a fermentation process and used to make the molecular scaffold for the drug. David Reddy, the New Zealand biochemist who heads Tamiflu production and sales for Roche, explains: 'To extract this, we have to work in special fermentation tunnels which are the size of two double-deckers. The acid goes through different processes, but it is potentially highly explosive so the complexity is such that very few places in the world can actually do that stage. It makes it all slower because we have to work on it in small amounts so that we can control it. The product at this point is as toxic as cyanide.'

'How much would you pay for a packet of ten tiny capsules that might end up saving your life in a flu pandemic?'

Once the acid has been modified, it becomes inert. After that a voluminous, fluffy white powder is produced. 'It looks rather like newly formed snow,' comments Mr Reddy. 'But because it forms clumps we have to mix it with large amounts of alcohol to make it into small granules.' This part of production is often contracted out elsewhere, so Roche can speed up the ten-stage manufacturing process.

First licensed as a flu treatment back in 1998, oseltamivir was never initially seen as a big earner. The drug was mainly initially intended to protect mostly the vulnerable and the elderly from the most common strains of flu. In normal, seasonal flu, it reduces the time you have to take off work by one day. For years, Roche has struggled to persuade countries to buy the drug in order to treat normal flu, arguing that influenza is a considerable cause of death in the West and the drug has a good safety record. But then along came H5N1 and suddenly, they no longer had to make the argument. Their dilemma now is how to make much more of it, while clinging onto the right to be the sole manufacturer.

THE NEGLECTED WEAPON

Tamiflu is not the only drug that may help in combating bird flu. There is another anti-viral medication known as Relenza, or zanamivir. Both Tamiflu and Relenza belong to a class of drug known as neuraminidase inhibitors. They work by closing the door on the virus, even when the infection is already inside the body. The drugs inhibit, or prevent, the neuraminidase enzyme – the spikes sticking out of the virus's coat – from being able to move from one cell into another, and spreading throughout the lungs. (See page 28 for more about neuraminidase.)

'It's a really clever mechanism because by stopping the infection in its tracks, it relieves symptoms without affecting many other organs. '

It's a really clever mechanism because by stopping the infection in its tracks, it relieves symptoms without affecting many other organs. The drugs, developed in the 1990s, are both safe and well-tolerated and they have now been used on many millions of patients worldwide to relieve normal influenza symptoms.

However, Relenza is a less popular choice for stockpiling, because instead of being taken orally as a capsule, it has to be inhaled through the mouth using a handheld device. Doctors worry that some patients might not be able to use it correctly, especially if they have intellectual or co-ordination impairments, however for the majority of adults it is a viable option.

Some researchers think that Relenza, made by GlaxoSmithKline, should also be stockpiled, along with Tamiflu, because it could give government another important weapon in the fight against an outbreak. In a commentary in the *Lancet* medical journal, Kenneth Tsang, from the University of Hong Kong, wrote in August 2005 that it is not enough to rely on Tamiflu alone. He also called for clinical trials combining Relenza and Tamiflu to see if the combination works better than either drug alone. He wrote: 'A vaccine for H5N1 will not be available in the foreseeable months. Even if pharmaceutical manufacturing begins soon after an outbreak, there would not be sufficient supply for the countries most in need, i.e. the Asian nations.' And he suggested that perhaps the manufacturing of the vaccine and the neuraminidase inhibitors should begin in Asia.

Countries are divided on this, however. America is stockpiling Relenza, while the UK has decided not to do so, relying instead on Tamiflu backed up by vaccines when they are eventually made.

Tamiflu dosage:

To be really effective, it has to be taken within 48 hours of the first flu symptoms appearing and a normal treatment course is two 75mg capsules a day, for five days. It can also be taken preventively to reduce the risk of catching the disease in the first place. For this preventive (or prophylactic) use, patients must be aged over thirteen, and they should take one tablet a day, for as long as they may be exposed to the virus.

It can also be given as 'post-exposure prophylaxis'. If a member of your family succumbed to the virus, you might be given Tamiflu to lower your chances of being infected. In this case, you would take one 75mg capsule daily for at least seven days following contact with the flu, and for up to six weeks if there was an outbreak in the community.

Women who are pregnant cannot take Tamiflu because of possible harm to the unborn child. The drug is not licensed for babies under the age of one.

(*continued over*)

Relenza dosage:

Again, treatment should be started within two days of the first symptoms to be most effective. A special inhaler is placed in the mouth and the medication is inhaled directly into the air passages and lungs. Patients need to have two puffs of the inhaler in the morning and two in the evening for five days. It can also work as a preventive medication.

Women who are breastfeeding or pregnant should not use it. Asthmatics or those with chronic bronchitis may also not be able to use this inhaler. It is not licensed for use in children under the age of twelve and should be used with caution by anyone who has an unstable chronic illness or a compromised immune system.

WHY THE DRUGS MIGHT HELP IN A PANDEMIC

There are a number of uncertainties about how anti-viral medication would work if H5N1 mutated to become a humanized strain. No pharmaceutical company would ever be allowed to carry out a clinical trial where you infected healthy human volunteers with a lethal virus like H5N1 and then gave half of them Tamiflu, half a placebo, and studied the results. The only way in which we can guess at the reduction of mortality rates it might achieve is by conducting studies on animals.

Avian influenza expert Dr Robert Webster and his colleagues at the St Jude Children's Research Hospital in Memphis, Tennessee, carried out a clinical trial with Tamiflu. They found that out of 80 mice infected with H5N1, those that received the drug soon after symptoms appeared had an 80 per cent survival rate. Without it, all of them died. But the timing is crucial. The survival rate fell to only 50 per cent in the mice trials if they were given it five days after symptoms appeared.

Many of the people who have so far died in Asia after contracting the disease from chickens have not received the drug at an early stage. In many countries, it is difficult to correctly diagnose the symptoms of flu and then get the medication to the patient within a 48-hour period. Dr Jeremy Farrar, who works at the Hospital for Tropical Diseases in Vietnam's Ho Chi Minh City, says that with the patients he has seen, the initial symptoms are just like many other kinds of illness, and it is extremely difficult to pick out people who might need the medication. 'It's a horrible infection as it develops, but in the early phase, when you are most infectious, it's just a fever and a cough, and millions of people in Asia have that every day of the week. It's not easy to distinguish from other illnesses.'

As someone on the front line, who has treated patients with H5N1, he is not convinced that the drug is quite as magical as it's made out to be. He told me: 'Oseltamivir is important for us but we shouldn't exaggerate the benefits. Even with common or garden flu, it only reduces the days off work by one day, and it may not reduce mortality.'

'They found that out of 80 mice infected with H5N1, those that received the drug soon after symptoms appeared had an 80 per cent survival rate.'

The data so far shows that Tamiflu produces a 38 per cent reduction in the severity of symptoms of normal flu, and a 67 per cent reduction in secondary complications such as bronchitis, pneumonia and sinusitis. However, there are concerns that the drug may not work as well if H5N1 mutates and changes its genetic make-up. Although it would still target the neuraminidase protein sticking out of the flu virus, other genetic changes to the virus may render it less effective.

Experts are worried that resistance to Tamiflu and Relenza could build up if they are too widely taken in communities as bird flu is becoming a human strain. In the case of one Vietnamese girl infected with the lethal form of H5N1, Tamiflu failed to work and researchers found that the virus in her body had become resistant to the drug. Everyone knew that this was always a risk but the fact that it has already happened is a real blow.

Yoshiro Kawaoka and his colleagues from Tokyo University reported in *Nature* on 14 October 2005 that the girl did recover, but not because of the drug. They carried out tests on ferrets, a creature that is often used in such research, and found one piece of good news – that the virus was still sensitive to Relenza. Kawaoka wrote that the case 'raises the concern that oseltamivir may not be sufficient to fight a potential H5N1 pandemic'. If a resistant strain of the flu became widespread, Tamiflu might not be much use.

Another worry about Tamiflu arose in November 2005, also from Japan, the country that uses more of the drug than any other for normal flu each year. Doctors reported that there were fears it might be linked to suicidal behaviour, after two teenagers who had been on the drug for flu treatment killed themselves. The connection between Tamiflu and possible psychological side effects was made by Dr Rokuro Hama, the head of the Japan Institute for Pharmacovigilance. Drug safety regulators in the US and Europe immediately reviewed its safety among children and adolescents to see if there was any danger of serious psychiatric disorders. In November 2005, the US Food and Drug Administration (FDA) reported they had found no evidence it caused psychiatric harm.

THE ROW OVER WHO SHOULD MAKE THE DRUG

Roche has increasingly come under pressure to relax its patent on Tamiflu. A patent gives the manufacturer the right, for a limited amount of time, to stop others from making or selling a new therapy. Some large companies that manufacture generic drugs (where the patent has come to an end) have announced their intentions to produce it, arguing that their countries cannot afford to buy it at current prices.

It's very unusual for a drug company to relax the patent on any drug, particularly one that is making them such a vast sum of money. In the third quarter of last year, Roche posted profits of 859 million Swiss francs (around £378 million) – an astonishing result, which meant its share price leapt up. The rise was almost wholly due to the insatiable demand for Tamiflu. However, under new laws poorer nations now have the right to issue compulsory licences that would allow their own manufacturers to make a medication if they can show that the human need for it is overwhelming.

At a press conference held by Roche in its Basel headquarters in November 2005, William Burns, the chief executive of the company's pharmaceuticals division, made it quite clear that they were not going to relax the patents on the drug. He explained that patents are society's way of rewarding innovation, and he reiterated a commonly held view among pharmaceutical giants that if there were no patents, there would simply be no new drugs in the world, because the profit motive would disappear overnight.

The Swiss-based company, under enormous political pressure, has begun talking to manufacturers in poorer countries to see if they could run at least part of the manufacturing process to reduce costs. It's not hard to see why Vietnam and others might want to make their own medicine. Roche's very cheapest price for Tamiflu, when it is selling it to a government in powder form, not capsules, is still 7€ per treatment course (ten capsules). That's £4.95 sterling, or $8.23 US at current exchange rates (end of 2005). For some nations, stockpiling it at that price would absorb their entire health budget for the year.

'...under new laws poorer nations now have the right to issue compulsory licences that would allow their own manufacturers to make a medication if they can show that the human need for it is overwhelming. '

Some countries are pressing ahead with plans to make their own versions of Tamiflu. In November 2005, the Chinese government, faced with several outbreaks of the H5N1 virus in its poultry, announced its intention to manufacture the drug using its own scientists. There are likely to be other challenges to Roche's position in 2006, and some new drugs aimed at disabling many different strains of flu are already in the pipeline.

THE SIZE OF GOVERNMENT STOCKPILES

Different governments have made their own decisions about how much Tamiflu to stockpile for the needs of their population (see page 96). The figures are changing every month but what is clear is that some governments began to plan ahead far earlier than others what they were going to need. Back in 2004 the British

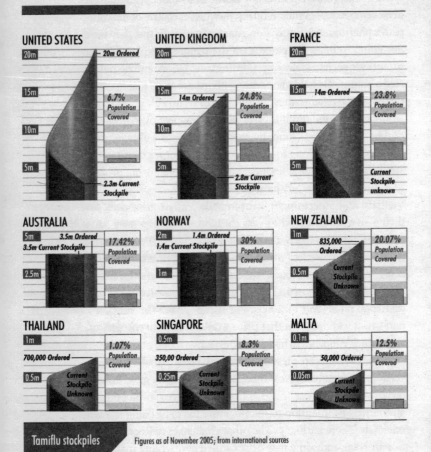

UNITED STATES
20m Ordered
6.7% Population Covered
2.3m Current Stockpile

UNITED KINGDOM
14m Ordered
24.8% Population Covered
2.8m Current Stockpile

FRANCE
14m Ordered
23.8% Population Covered
Current Stockpile unknown

AUSTRALIA
3.5m Ordered
3.5m Current Stockpile
17.42% Population Covered

NORWAY
1.4m Ordered
1.4m Current Stockpile
30% Population Covered

NEW ZEALAND
835,000 Ordered
Current Stockpile Unknown
20.07% Population Covered

THAILAND
700,000 Ordered
Current Stockpile Unknown
1.07% Population Covered

SINGAPORE
350,00 Ordered
Current Stockpile Unknown
8.3% Population Covered

MALTA
50,000 Ordered
Current Stockpile Unknown
12.5% Population Covered

Tamiflu stockpiles — Figures as of November 2005; from international sources

government ordered enough of the drug from Roche to cover a quarter of its population, but the complete amount won't arrive until September 2006. However, the US has only ordered enough to cover 6.7 per cent of its population. (See pages 109–112 for more on the US's preparations.)

COUNTERFEIT DRUGS

The Internet – with its lack of security and checks – makes it easy to peddle fake drugs, sometimes at enormous cost. It has long provided a marketplace for ruthless gangs who make millions of dollars each year producing counterfeit medications. At the moment most of these medications end up in the developing world, but they are increasingly becoming sophisticated operations capable of infiltrating the markets in Europe and America.

Many thousands of courses of Tamiflu have been sold over the Internet, since demand took off in the autumn of 2005. Before then it was possible to get the drug from the chemist (with a prescription) or buy it in pharmacies abroad. At present, stocks are so low that people have been turning to the Internet. However, it is not a good idea to buy medication of any kind off the Internet, because its source is unknown.

Roche has already come across the first packet of fake Tamiflu. Although there are few clear details, their experts say they found a packet of ten capsules which had originated in South Africa. According to Eugene Tierney, global head of virology and transplantation at Roche, the outside packaging was perfect – indistinguishable from the real thing. 'But when you opened it up, you could see that the blister pack [the packaging material for the drug] was not the same at all. Even the capsules looked different.' When they tested it, the active ingredient was completely missing from the capsule, so it would have been useless against influenza.

If you are tempted to buy a medication over the net, how can you tell if it is real or fake? These are the things to look out for:

- Check the colour of the capsules. With Tamiflu, they should be half yellow, half light grey.

- Look at the batch number and the code which is printed on the foil of the blister pack. This should match the numbers printed on the outside of the packet.

- If in doubt, ring up the manufacturer. They may ask you to send it in and they will check it for you.

Counterfeit drugs could contain dangerous chemicals and consumers would have no way of knowing that beforehand. As with any medication, it is important to talk to your doctor before taking them to check that they won't react with any other medication you might be taking. Buying drugs on the net is a gamble – and do you really want to gamble with your health?

THE REAL HOPE – A VACCINE

The single most important response to a bird flu pandemic would be the creation of an effective vaccine. This is the only medication that will give long-term protection, and by far the easiest method of covering an entire population. Vaccines made to counteract particular strains of flu tend to be long-lasting and effective. Economically, they make sense too; once the initial high costs of developing the vaccine have been met, the production costs are usually cheap enough to make coverage of an entire population affordable.

'Vaccines harness the body's own ability to fight disease by triggering a response in the immune system.'

Each year, roughly 100 million doses of flu vaccine are made to protect nations around the world against the different flu strains in circulation. These inoculations against seasonal flu have already saved many thousands of people from a disease which, even in a normal year, can be lethal.

Vaccines harness the body's own ability to fight disease by triggering a response in the immune system. Each vaccine contains an antigen (a part of the virus's foreign protein) which will stimulate an immune reaction in the form of antibodies. When you are vaccinated, you receive a dose of the antigen that has been altered so that it is harmless, but your immune system still sends out its antibodies to fight the invader. When you are then actually exposed to the real, live virus, your body will already have the necessary antibodies to fight it off.

Unlike other diseases, such as measles, where you only need one shot to protect you for a lifetime, with flu you need a different vaccine each year because the virus changes so quickly. In normal years, the most difficult question for scientists is which particular strains of flu they should include in that year's virus. They usually take three strains which are different enough from those that have been around in previous years to attract attention.

The laboratories that do the preparatory work, such as the National Institute for Biological Standards and Controls in Hertfordshire, or the US Center for Disease Control and Prevention in Atlanta, Georgia, receive samples from around the world and log them in a database that shows where the strain came from, whether it caused serious illness and whether it is spreading rapidly.

A 'fingerprint' is then made showing the virus's genotype, and this is compared with other strains. They are stored in a deep freeze, and parts of the virus are grown either in eggs or in a special cell culture to be studied further. This is known as 'seeding' the virus.

'For reasons that are not fully understood, some flu strains are just much faster than others.'

If the coat protein looks new enough to cause trouble, scientists will test to see how infectious it is, and how quickly the immune system will respond to it. Meanwhile, researchers stay in constant touch with colleagues in different parts of the world to check which strains are spreading quickly. For reasons that are not fully understood, some flu strains are just much faster than others.

Once a decision has been made on which strains to use to make a vaccination, the rush is on. For normal seasonal flu, vaccines are made using eggs, a technique that was developed in the 1950s. This is a slow process, though. Eggs take weeks to grow, and they have to be specially produced to ensure that the supply is safe and clean.

Viral strains are injected into millions of fertilized chicken eggs and incubated there. The eggs are then opened and the virus is extracted and purified. The virus is treated chemically to kill it, while preserving the normal shape of the coat's proteins. Each final dose of vaccine is very small, containing barely fifteen-millionths of a gram of each of the three different strains, but they are enough to trigger an immunological defence.

Stephen Inglis, of the National Institute for Biological Standards and Controls, explains: 'Ours is one of a handful of laboratories authorized to make the seed strains for pandemic flu. It's our job to turn the dangerous strains into strains that can be changed by manufacturers into vaccine. We use a specific method, known as reverse genetics. This involves picking apart the genes of the virus and creating a new one, entirely from scratch. We load it up with the genes that code for the outside part of the virus, but we have taken out some of the lethal parts from the inside. This means that the human immune system can recognize it and attack it, but the most dangerous parts are no longer there.'

'The problem is that it will take between four and six months to make a vaccine once the disease has become fully human.'

So why don't we have a bird flu vaccine yet? The great problem lies in the timing. What the world needs is an inoculation that will work once the virus mutates to become a pandemic form, capable of spreading quickly between people. But to do this, scientists have to know the exact genotype of the strain. If one is made today on the basis of what we currently know about H5N1, it may not prove to be a good match in six months' time, or whenever it mutates. Guesswork doesn't mean much with vaccines.

Researchers have already isolated the material from the current viruses that people have caught from chickens in Southeast Asia, and this is being investigated. Some experts believe we should be using the genotype currently circulating to make a vaccine which might give us some limited immunity when the new 'humanized' form emerges. But others feel that it could be a waste of money and effort, given that it might not work at all for the next pandemic, if the virus has mutated a great deal from the subtype currently circulating.

The problem is that it will take between four and six months to make a vaccine once the disease has become fully human. Given that the outbreaks could spread around the world within one to two months, it is clear that there will not be enough vaccine ready to protect people in time for a pandemic, unless the disease spreads more slowly than is being predicted.

The good news, however, is that the pandemic threat has spurred several organizations and governments to start investing far more in vaccine development. Several 'prototype' vaccines are currently being looked at. The concept, heavily backed by leading American researchers, is that the science community should go as far down the road as possible in making a vaccine to overcome the initial regulatory hurdles, so that when we do have the right strain, the correct genetic material can be added at the final stage, and the vaccine will then be ready to go.

You could argue that the one good thing to be emerging from all the plans for a pandemic is the fact that world leaders have belatedly decided to do more to invest in vaccine technology. The question is: can the right shot be made in time?

'In a normal shot it [the flu inoculation] would have a cocktail of three haemagglutinin proteins, but in this it has just one – H5.'

TESTING THE NEW VACCINES

Who would volunteer to be a guinea pig for a new flu vaccine? Vic Maslanka for one – he was one of 150 adults to have taken part in a study at three American research centres to see if a new vaccine is safe, and whether it successfully triggers some kind of immune response.

The new experimental shot is nearly identical to the one which millions of people get every year, but it has one big difference. The key ingredient in any flu inoculation is the haemagglutinin protein which allows it to latch onto human cells. In a normal shot it would have a cocktail of three haemagglutinin proteins, but in this it has just one – H5.

Maslanka and the other volunteers were injected with different concentration of vaccines or just a saltwater placebo. Researchers then took blood tests every few months to see what levels of antibodies they had created against the H5 protein. The standard flu jab contains around 45 micrograms of haemagglutinin, and researchers want to know whether they need a lot more of it or a lot less to get antibody production.

Maslanka, an engineer, is glad to be helping. He remembers when he was a child mowing the grass in a cemetery, and many of the headstones bore the same date – 1918. His parents later told him that the Spanish flu had killed many millions of people around the globe that year. Two of them were his own relatives, he discovered. So when he heard that the University of Maryland School of Medicine was preparing to test a vaccine designed to prevent the next pandemic, he signed up. 'This was personal,' he explained.

There had been hopes for a hybrid vaccine, which has already gone through one clinical trial. America's National Institutes of Health paid Sanofi Pasteur, a French vaccine manufacturer, and Chiron, a manufacturer based in California, to produce hybrid vaccines. They came up with some interesting results, showing that each person would need two 90-microgram doses of the antigen, the viral protein that forms the basis for the vaccine. But at the current rate of production worldwide, that means that there would only be enough vaccine for 75 million people – just – around a quarter of the US population.

Another solution researchers have been looking at is to boost the power of each shot. This can be done by combining them with a simple chemical known as an 'adjuvant', which stimulates the immune system by making the vaccine linger at the site where it has been injected. GlaxoSmithKline's German firm has made such a vaccine, and it appears to give full immunity against relatives of the H5 family with two doses, at just 1.9 micrograms each.

Trials of the adjuvant vaccines are beginning, looking at doses down to 7.5 micrograms, and these are planned in the next year for Canada, the US and Japan. But in order to protect as many people as possible with a limited supply, we must try to find the very lowest dose that might be needed, according to David Fedson, founder of the vaccine industry's pandemic task force. 'By not determining the lowest dose that is acceptably immunogenic, the vaccine companies have shown they do not understand the unforgiving arithmetic of pandemic vaccine supply,' Fedson told the *New Scientist* magazine in October 2005. 'That means millions will not receive the vaccine, and thousands will die. Economists call this an opportunity cost. I call it a tragedy.'

Adjuvant vaccines may be the solution. After the 1997 outbreak of bird flu in Hong Kong, one group of people were given an adjuvant dose and a study published in 2005 in the *Journal of Infections* showed that years later, they still had significant immunity to the strain of flu that is currently circulating.

But there can be drawbacks too. Some adjuvants can cause a mild reaction at the site of the injection, and they are only licensed for use in flu vaccines in twenty countries. Rino Rappuoli , the chief scientific officer of Chiron, is working on one in Italy, where 18 million people have been treated with the adjuvanted vaccine for normal flu. He believes that if adjuvants could allow doctors to give half the normal flu dose – and thus double the amount available – you get a much better immune response.

BRITAIN'S RESPONSE

Britain has ordered 2 million doses of a vaccine made using the current H5N1 strain. But it has also ordered 120 million doses of a vaccine to be made when the virus becomes humanized. As every person will need two shots for full immunity, the order is big enough to cover everyone in the country. (See Chapter 7 for more on Britain's preparations.) Sir Liam Donaldson, the UK's chief medical officer, spelled out the problems at a briefing to London journalists back in October 2004.

'We obviously face a choice about whether to purchase the vaccine in which the present strains of H5N1 are used. The Americans have tried to do this but the first generation vaccines [using the current strain] were not that effective – they didn't provoke an immune response. We have now ordered some of it –

2 million doses as a contingency – which will be ready next year, and this might be useful for healthcare workers.'

He continued: 'The truth is that we can't have the perfect vaccine before we know exactly what the strain of the virus is. Once the virus becomes "humanized", when it is easily transmitted from person to person, that is when it can cause a pandemic. Each virus has its own signature, and we have to identify that before we can have the right immunization programme.'

WHY VACCINES HAVE FALLEN INTO NEGLECT

What is really needed is a new form of vaccine technology. It's not an area that interests the big pharmaceutical companies much because the profits are uncertain and the demands are unpredictable. But a lot of experts want to see the governments giving researchers more financial incentives for coming up with new ideas so that we could target these evolving viruses.

'Each virus has its own signature, and we have to identify that before we can have the right immunization programme.'

One of the world's leading experts is Dr Anthony Fauci, head of the National Institute of Allergy and Infectious Diseases, America's leading research organization in this field. When I spoke to him, he was frustrated at the lack of action to improve vaccine development – although since then President Bush has announced far more funding for initiatives.

Dr Fauci told me: 'The really limiting factor is the global capacity to manufacture vaccine. This has been a smouldering problem for years, and we face it annually with seasonal influenza. People don't realize it, but it causes significant mortality, and in the States alone is responsible for 36,000 deaths a year.

'When we go into a pandemic, the numbers can obviously go into millions. But every year, vaccine manufacturing is never fully addressed because people don't generally perceive flu as a threat.'

Dr Fauci said that the vaccine they have worked on did produce a reasonable immune response, 'but it requires a much higher dose than we thought...There's no shortage of good science to make a seed virus for the vaccine but capacity is a big problem.'

And behind it all lies the indisputable fact that for years, it has been more profitable for pharmaceutical companies to manufacture drugs for 'lifestyle' problems, such as obesity, than it has to make one for an infection. As Fauci put it: 'If you're a company executive and you could make a new kind of Viagra, or a lipid-lowering drug for $200 million, why would you go for a vaccine instead, where the risk and the costs are so high?'

Nevertheless, the increasing worries about a pandemic strain have forced governments to start investing in vaccines. Back in September 2005, Sanofi Pasteur, part of the Sanofi-Aventis group, won a $100 million contract to supply the United States with a vaccine against H5N1, part of their plan to stockpile 20 million doses of vaccine. But will it just be the richest countries that are able to afford to do this?

As Dr Hitoshi Oshitani, the World Health Organization's Asian communicable diseases expert, has warned, the early vaccines are unlikely to protect against an emerging pandemic virus. He also fears that once a pandemic occurs, the world's richest nations may dominate vaccine supply. 'The distribution of a vaccine will be a major issue when a pandemic starts. There is no mechanism for distribution,' he said. Asked whether poorer Asian nations such as Cambodia and Vietnam would get a vaccine, Dr Oshitani replied: 'Probably not.'

6 THE WORLD PLAYS CATCH UP

'The success of dealing with avian influenza and a human pandemic depends entirely on the extent to which countries, scientists and health organizations are going to be able to work together across continents and between countries. The preparedness of the world depends not so much on who is strong, but on who is weak.'

Dr David Nabarro   Senior United Nation System Coordinator for Avian and Human Influenza

Faced with a biological disaster as potentially devastating as bird flu, the need for countries to work together and share their resources has never been greater. After the harrowing near-miss of the SARS epidemic in 2003, the world is looking once more at the possibility that a lethal pathogen could cross borders and infect large areas of the world within days, while there is no effective medical remedy to hand.

Some nations – and several international organizations – woke up to the problem long before others. Right through 2004, when bird flu was insidiously working its way into poultry populations across the Far East, many

Western countries saw it as a very distant threat. The US, in particular, ignored the problem. The European Union also admits that it did not do enough to help Vietnam or Thailand eradicate the disease at an early stage.

By the autumn of 2005, it became clear that bird flu was now endemic in millions of birds in Asia and it has arrived on Europe's doorstep, with infected birds found in Turkey, Croatia, Greece and Romania. What will the world do now that H5N1 has gained a foothold across a large area of the globe? Different countries have different priorities for tackling the infection, but there are no quick or easy answers.

'The US has been badly prepared for pandemics in the past, and several American presidents have been caught out.'

In October 2005 Professor Colin Blakemore, director-general of the UK's Medical Research Council, visited China with a team of influenza experts to see for himself the scale of the problems. He told me: 'This is a really horrible disease. What we've seen in the people who are infected is that they die really quickly. They get a raging pneumonia that just dissolves the lungs, and then it can affect the kidneys and the brain.

'We need to know far more about the disease in humans. How are people becoming infected? We think it's mostly airborne infection but it's not clear.

'To me, the most important priority should be more surveillance in the field. The big worry is the silent infections that can be carried in ducks or geese. We need to know the scale of the infection in these birds, and that is a massive undertaking. But we also need more surveillance of people, so that it can be detected at a much earlier stage. That's hard in a country like China where so many people have no access to a doctor, and live miles away from a hospital.'

The British response to the threat of bird flu is described in Chapter 7, but in this chapter I'll look at the reactions and level of preparedness in some other countries around the world, as well as major global organizations like the World Bank and the World Health Organization.

THE PREDICAMENT FACING THE US

The US has been badly prepared for pandemics in the past, and several American presidents have been caught out. Woodrow Wilson found himself in difficulty back in 1918 when the Spanish flu pandemic was at its height. He ignored the advice of senior military doctors and kept sending shipments of troops abroad on crowded vessels, which came to be known as 'death ships'. The high mortality rates as a result of influenza, combined with riots in the army camps caused by a severe shortage of food, did him great political damage. He was to catch pandemic flu himself in 1919, but survived the experience.

Six decades later, President Gerald Ford came badly unstuck thanks to flu. In 1976, his officials convinced him that there might be a serious epidemic of the disease that winter as a new strain was circulating in pigs. He ordered the production of millions of doses of extra flu vaccine, but the companies manufacturing it insisted that

'Some experts believe that the events of 9/11 were so cataclysmic for America that all their resources were focused on the threat of terrorism...'

they had to have special liability protection, so Congress passed a law making the government bear all liability. They ended up with a bill for $90 million when lawsuits were brought by individuals who had suffered a rare paralytic complication of the vaccine. And there was no flu epidemic after all.

Is this recent history a reason why the US has responded so late to the current threat of a pandemic? Others would point to more recent events. Some experts believe that the events of 9/11 were so cataclysmic for America that all their resources have been focused on the threat of terrorism, and in particular the possibility of new biological weapons being developed. Policy-makers have ignored all the other warnings that were coming their way, including that of a flu pandemic.

The devastation caused by hurricanes Katrina and Rita in September 2005 was a wake-up call for Washington, revealing to the administration that when a natural disaster strikes, you need to have a plan in place to deal with it. Following the damage done to New Orleans, President Bush looked again at the US strategy for dealing with a flu pandemic and found that they didn't really have one that was realistic.

The president had reason to be worried. A draft document outlining the administration's ability to cope with a pandemic flu outbreak revealed that the country was woefully unprepared. The document, leaked to the *New York Times* at the beginning of October 2005, spelled out the harsh facts: hospitals would be overwhelmed, riots would engulf vaccination clinics and food would be in short supply. In a worst-case scenario, more than 1.9 million Americans would die, and 8.5 million would be hospitalized. The bill would come to more than $450 billion.

It is little wonder, then, that in the autumn of 2005 the president called the leaders of the nation's six top vaccine producers to the White House to explain to him how they could increase their vaccine capacity. They in turn spelled out to him that there were no quick fixes: it would mean millions of dollars of investment, but a vaccine that worked would be the only long-term defence against a lethal form of flu.

'It is a very ominous situation for the globe,' says Dr Julie L. Gerberding, director of the Center for Disease Control and Prevention in Atlanta, the US government body responsible for public health. The predictions for a pandemic in the US certainly look very bad. The Center for Disease Control predicts that a medium-level epidemic could kill up to 207,000 people. Initially, the Bush administration planned to have no more than 2.3 million treatments of anti-viral medication for their stockpile, which is not even enough to cover 1 per cent of the population. That amount has now been pushed up to 20 million doses of the anti-viral medication, and a further 20 million doses of vaccine.

'We're way behind,' said Dr Jeffrey Levi, a policy advisor at the non-profit organization Trust for America's Health. 'The United States cannot come close to the UK's 25 per cent level. For us, that would be at least 75 million treatments. We have to hope that the pandemic doesn't strike before we've ordered enough and received enough that it will provide some kind of protection.'

Politically, the US has had little sympathy with the efforts of Asian countries to tackle the risks, and the Bush administration has made clear its dislike of the UN system, further hampering efforts to co-ordinate their approach. Although they have some of the world's leading experts in the field of influenza, and have poured enormous amounts of money into research on viruses, there appears to be little interest from the White House in assisting those battling against the disease on the front line.

Laurie Garrett, an award-winning journalist, commented recently that it was difficult for America to make multinational agreements on how to tackle the pandemic risk when Congress was full of members who openly criticised China and Vietnam. 'It's China with whom we need to be collaborating on this. And it's hard when you have some members of Congress who still think of Vietnam as the enemy, as if we were still fighting the Vietnam War.'

'...it's hard when you have some members of Congress who still think of Vietnam as the enemy, as if we were still fighting the Vietnam War.'

Others want to see Congress doing more to lead the international community to take decisive action, particularly by establishing a set of incentives that would encourage nations to report flu outbreaks quickly and fully.

Writing in the *New York Times*, Democrat Barak Obama, a member of the Senate Foreign Relations Committee, and Republican Richard Lugar, its chairman, stated: 'So far H5N1 has not been found in the United States. But in an age when you can board planes in Bangkok or Hong Kong and arrive in Chicago, Indianapolis or New York in hours, we must face the reality that these killer diseases are not isolated health problems half a world away, but direct and immediate threats to security and prosperity here at home.'

By 1 November 2005 the president was meeting experts at the US National Institutes of Health in Maryland, unveiling a $7 billion strategy to show how seriously he was taking the threat. 'Avian flu has developed some of the characteristics needed to cause a pandemic,' he told his audience. 'If the virus developed the capacity for sustained human-to-human transmission, it could spread quickly around the world.'

But the stakes are very high. As hurricanes have shown, the US is not that well prepared to deal with natural disasters, and the president must now be wondering if, like his predecessors, he will also be caught out by influenza.

THE CANADIAN RESPONSE

How will we know when a new pandemic strain of flu emerges? Even if it occurs in Southeast Asia, the first signs may be detected thousands of miles away in Canada, because the Canadians were far-sighted enough back in 2004 to set up a global system which tracks emerging diseases as they develop.

'...the first signs may be detected thousands of miles away in Canada...'

The Global Public Health Intelligence Network, based in Ottawa, sifts through media reports, radio broadcasts and websites from around the world and transmits relevant information about potential threats immediately in six languages. Alerts are triggered by more than 30,000 key words which could indicate a disease outbreak and the computer system then contacts the World Health Organization, who investigate the threat.

The programme was developed by the Public Health Agency of Canada, and is managed by the Centre for Emergency Preparedness and Response, the body which had to deal with the SARS outbreak of 2003. Dr Ron St John, its director-general, says the programme has some interesting features. 'It's remarkable that you can receive something written in Chinese characters and one minute later it's in English, French, Spanish, Arabic and Russian,' he said.

As one example of why early warning is so important, the Chinese government first reported the disease that would become known as SARS to the WHO on 11 February, 2003. However, the disease is believed to have started in China's Guangdong province in November 2002. If there had been such a tracking system in existence at the time, it would have picked up early mentions of a new illness in the local press and might have kept SARS from spreading so far around the globe.

Canada is well prepared for a flu pandemic, and was one of the first countries to produce a plan. It intends to have enough doses of Tamiflu for 4 million people and has set out clearly how it will prioritize those who receive treatment. It also intends to stockpile Relenza, but the government hasn't yet anounced how much they want. The government has also held a full public consultation over health measures that may work, asking people to write in about their priorities and such issues as effective hygiene control. Ministers have been pushing other nations to do far more to protect against a pandemic, and Canada has set up a $15 million programme with the Far East to increase surveillance there.

AUSTRALIA BRACES ITSELF

Australia is wracked with anxiety over avian influenza. The topic is constantly on the news, which is hardly surprising given its proximity to Southeast Asia. The fact that Australia is on the flight-path for many birds migrating south from Vietnam and Indonesia does not fill the Australians with optimism.

So far, very little firm advice has been offered to Australian citizens. Professor Marie-Louise McLaws, an associate professor at the University of New South Wales in Sydney who advises the World Health Organization on surveillance of epidemics, is disappointed that her government has not done more to give the public solid information. 'A lot of the people who work for the Department of Health don't want to talk openly about it. The average Australian is not being told in much detail exactly what is happening,' said Professor McLaws, whose work includes research on the emergence of SARS. 'People are being told about the problems with Tamiflu, such as resistance, and they are being told about the stockpiling. But we don't know yet who is going to receive it prophylactically [as a preventive measure].'

In fact, the truth is that Australia is much better prepared for a pandemic than many other countries. Its government has stockpiled both drugs and the equipment that would be needed in a pandemic. Hospitals have negative pressure units (sealed areas kept below normal air pressure), which are the best way of isolating highly infectious patients. In order to prevent bird flu being brought into the country, they have introduced thermal scanners to screen travellers on arrival and pinpoint any who have a raised temperature.

Two vaccine producers have been contracted to ensure sufficient pandemic vaccine will be available for every citizen, and its surveillance systems have been boosted as part of a programme costing 156 million Australian dollars.

' In order to prevent bird flu being brought into the country, they have introduced thermal scanners to screen travellers on arrival and pinpoint any who have a raised temperature.'

Currently, they are most worried about H5N1-infected birds being imported, as well as geese which might migrate into the country from the north. In October 2005, Australia banned imports of birds from Canada after three pigeons certified as healthy by Canadian officials tested positive for avian flu antibodies while in quarantine. This led to much questioning about their quarantine procedures, but on the whole Australia is one of the better-prepared countries. They know that when a pandemic strain emerges, they are likely to be hit at an early stage simply because of their geographical proximity to the worst-affected countries.

JAPAN'S ACTION PLAN

Japan is taking the threat of a pandemic extremely seriously. The country has had several outbreaks of H5N1 in its domestic poultry but moved swiftly to deal with it on each occasion. In November 2005, the Japanese government published a plan outlining how they would cope if there was an outbreak of a human version of bird flu. Once a widespread outbreak was confirmed but before it became a full-scale global pandemic, patients found to have the infection would be hospitalized, if necessary by force, schools would be closed in the infected areas and large public gatherings would be banned. Officials at the health ministry in Tokyo hope that these fairly restrictive public health measures would curb the spread of the disease, at least in the early stages.

Their action plan, based on the six phases of a pandemic outlined by the World Health Organization (see page 129), estimates that as many as 32 million Japanese could catch the disease, 2 million would be hospitalized and in the worst case scenario 640,000 could die if avian flu were to become transmissible between humans in the near future. They have started increasing their stockpile of Tamiflu and should have enough to cover 25 million people before the end of March 2007. That would provide a course for nearly one in five citizens, which is not as high a percentage as Britain, France or Norway but more than the US.

PREPARATIONS IN INDIA

India has not yet had a case of bird flu but millions of birds fly there from the Far East each year, so preparing for the threat is not easy. They do not have a high level of surveillance on farms in the countryside, but the Indian government is taking the threat very seriously.

One of their hopes is that they will be able to manufacture their own anti-viral medications, especially Tamiflu. Officials have said that under the present policy there is no bar to making the drug in India but generic companies who want to follow the same complex, ten-stage manufacturing process would have to seek permission from the manufacturer, Roche. (See pages 94–95, for more about the battle over who makes the drug.)

Three Indian companies – Cipla, Ranbaxy and Hetero – have stated that they are ready to manufacture the drugs. Malvinder Mohan Singh president of Ranbaxy's pharmaceuticals division said they know the company is capable of manufacturing the drug in lab scale. 'We are now preparing for commercial production. We have had discussions with Roche and are expecting a decision soon.'

Roche has indicated that it has received about 150 requests for licences to manufacture Tamiflu, and has already held discussions with eight possible partners. It expects to shortlist the candidates by December 2005.

STRIVING FOR SOLIDARITY IN EUROPE

European nations have watched bird flu drawing closer to them with a great deal of trepidation. Romania, Turkey, Croatia and Greece have found infected birds and immediately brought in stringent procedures to control the infection, but the sight of men in protective suits culling geese has not been a pleasant one. Although the disease is still in birds and has not infected a single human being in Europe, the public has reacted with alarm and started to question whether politicians are doing enough to combat the threat.

The ability of different European nations will be put to the test at the end of 2005, when an imaginary flu scenario is enacted by officials in command centres across Europe to see how they cope. No staff will be mobilized – it is a tabletop exercise designed to see where the weak points in the infrastructure might lie. For example, in the event of an emergency will all countries be able to communicate with the public about their health services at an early enough stage?

Some feel that Europe has not done enough to produce a co-ordinated plan stretching across borders, which could pick up the earliest infections in birds, as well as preparing for a human pandemic. Their tardiness in helping poorer nations tackle the threat was acknowledged by the EU's health commissioner Markos Kyprianou. Speaking in Vietnam at the start of a ten-day tour of Southeast Asia in November 2005, he admitted that the EU 'should have reacted more quickly to help Southeast Asia to tackle the problem.' But, he added: 'It's better late than never. The EU is interested in co-operating with Asia to solve the problem.'

Perhaps what is needed now is a financial commitment from the wealthier nations to contribute towards the cost of a pandemic. The European Commission is considering setting up a 'solidarity' fund of around 1 billion euros which would be used to buy anti-viral drugs, as well as vaccines. Such a move would have

La Ferme de la Vallée

As chicken and duck breeders, Michel Darcq and his wife Mireille face an uncertain future while France prepares to deal with bird flu. La Ferme de la Vallée (Valley Farm) lies in an idyllic spot near Monnai, in Normandy, but they have been told that all birds have to be brought indoors. That means the geese, hens, turkeys and pheasants may no longer roam around freely.

> *Michel explains: 'We have what you would call a traditional way of farming. All our two thousand poultry are out every morning and spend the day eating grass, hay and maize but also the peelings from carrots. The quality of our produce comes from the fact that the birds live outdoors. They are only in at night. If the hygiene measures become draconian to the point where we have to shut them in all day, we will stop rearing them for the time it takes.'*
>
> *The couple is worried that when hens have to be kept indoors all day, they can be susceptible to many other illnesses. Luckily they also rear pigs for pork so they can diversify, but it won't be easy. 'Battery hen farming would be completely against our philosophy,' Michel says simply.*

to be agreed by all 25 EU members, but could be used to help support those with a lower stockpile than others. But member states would still be expected to draw up their own healthcare plans for dealing with a pandemic.

The European Scientific Working Group on Influenza, a network of health organizations and flu experts from across the EU, have called for the creation of a European Influenza Task Force which would oversee vaccine development and the production of more anti-viral drugs, as well as making communication easier between countries and agencies. Its chairman, Professor Albert Osterhaus, wants to see a real-time monitoring system of viral infections in migratory birds, so that virologists and ornithologists could collaborate closely. 'This would provide an early warning system for the introduction of influenza viruses that may threaten poultry and eventually other animal species, including humans, from avian reservoirs.'

FRANCE

With a population the same as Britain's, France has revised its pandemic plan and asked for 40 million vaccine doses to be prepared. They have already distributed 50 million flu masks to hospitals and by early 2006, 200 million masks will be available to protect healthcare workers. In 21 *départements*, they have ordered all poultry to be kept indoors to avoid contagion from wild birds.

GERMANY

Bavaria has banned poultry markets at least until the end of 2005. The German government believes a pandemic strain could infect up to one third of the population. They currently have enough stock-piled anti-viral drugs to treat one in ten people.

ITALY

The Italians have ordered the compulsory labelling of all poultry to show where it was raised and the date and place of slaughter, partly to assuage nervous consumers. They have brought in extra vets to work with farmers. Police units which enforce the border controls have been increased, to try to stop birds being smuggled in.

USING COMPUTERS TO PREDICT THE COURSE OF PANDEMICS

Computers can be invaluable in helping scientists to understand the spread and pattern of disease, a field known as epidemiology. Their use is crucial when trying to understand the behaviour of such lethal viruses as bird flu.

Back in 2004, researchers from five different institutions set out to answer the question: 'Is it possible to stop an outbreak of human bird flu in its tracks once the virus mutates?' Their task was challenging to say the least, because until the highly pathogenic subtype becomes fully transmissible between people, scientists find it hard to predict how they will be able to contain the disease. Nevertheless, they examined the problem using computer programmes in centres based in five different time zones: London, Baltimore, Paris, Hong Kong, and the town of Nonthaburi in Thailand.

Professor Neil Ferguson, the youthful-looking professor of mathematical biology at London's Imperial College, was the lead researcher. He decided to simulate an outbreak in rural Thailand, assuming that a virulently pathogenic form of H5N1 had mutated to become highly contagious.

'Some of their findings were alarming. Computer modelling showed that to stop an outbreak, cases would have to be identified before there were more than 30 people who were infected.'

Working with researchers in the Nonthaburi area, they looked at the methods of transmission between people and how easily it might spread. Researchers then used computer modelling based on the population of 85 million Thai people to assess which methods of containment would work best.

Some of their findings were alarming. Computer modelling showed that to stop an outbreak, cases would have to be identified before there were more than 30 people who were infected. To limit the spread, anti-viral drugs would have to be given to 20,000 people closest to those who were infected in a very short space of time.

The research revealed that controlling an epidemic is increasingly difficult once more than 40 people have caught the disease, or once it has reached a major city. Closing schools and stopping people from travelling was important, but not nearly as important as detecting an outbreak at a very early stage.

In August 2005 Professor Ferguson told a packed press conference in London: 'Until now the idea of stopping a flu pandemic had not been investigated and what [our research] shows is that controlling a human outbreak is potentially feasible but only in the earliest stages. It is the only strategy which could have a dramatic impact on the levels of death and disease that a new pandemic would cause.'

He added; 'What we have shown is that if the virus is quickly transmissible we have a chance of stopping it but the control is challenging. We need to treat people quickly and detect people quickly, mostly through use of anti-virals and social distancing measures.'

But Ferguson's team did offer a ray of hope. They worked out that the reproductive number (RO) of bird flu – the number of people who would be infected by another person during the course of the illness – was not as high as expected. In the past, people have put the RO for flu at between four and ten. In fact, for humanized bird flu it is likely to be just two. The disease would be contagious, but not as contagious as measles, for example, which has an RO of fifteen.

> *'They worked out that the reproductive number (RO) of bird flu – the number of people who would be infected by another person during the course of the illness – was not as high as expected.'*

THE ECONOMIC COSTS OF A PANDEMIC

It is hard to over-estimate the amount of economic damage that could be done by a bird flu pandemic. The World Bank has warned that the effects are potentially so far-reaching that it could cost the global economy up to 2 per cent of its gross domestic product (GDP), some $800 billion (£458 billion) in all.

'It is fair to assume the shock during a flu epidemic could be even larger and last longer than SARS,' said Milan Brahmbhatt, World Bank chief economist for the Asia-Pacific region, speaking in November 2005. SARS caused widespread global panic before it was contained in 2003, and Far Eastern economies were badly hit at the time, but picked up again once the infection was controlled.

Early in 2005, the World Bank predicted that the threat of bird flu was a real one for Southeast Asia. 'One large shadow looms over the generally positive economic outlook we have sketched out... and that is avian flu,' predicted World Bank economist Homi Kharas.

The Bank has announced a $1billion emergency funding drive as a means of averting a catastrophe. They want to fund $500 million of grants to aid the countries in the front-line of any pandemic, and they hope to raise the same amount again through donations. The Bush administration has said that it will earmark around $251 million for pandemic planning in foreign countries, and has already given Southeast Asia around $30 million, much of it money that was originally intended for reconstruction after the tsunami.

But it is not only Asia that needs investment. It would cost at least $170 million to prepare Africa for the threat, by increasing its flu surveillance, equipping laboratories and training staff to control the disease in birds, while training health workers to treat people. There are an estimated 1.1 billion chickens in Africa, the vast majority of them kept outdoors where they have contact with wild birds, and the health services of the continent are already massively over-stretched, so any infection there could quickly snowball out of control.

PLANNING HOW TO WORK TOGETHER

The World Health Organization (WHO) was set up by the United Nations after World War II to improve the health of all nations – and their definition of health includes physical, mental and social wellbeing, rather than simply an absence of illness. Much of their work since then has involved combating infectious diseases, and their experts did extremely good work during the SARS outbreak of 2003, giving the world fresh information day by day and ensuring that hospitals knew how to enforce proper infection control. They issued their first warning about the threat of a bird flu pandemic during the 1997 outbreak in Hong Kong.

From the WHO's glass-fronted building set on a hill overlooking Geneva, officials have been working around the clock to keep track of H5N1 as well as preparing strategies for dealing with a potential human pandemic. This is what WHO is best at – giving governments fast, accurate advice on how to deal with emerging infections. They do so on a tiny budget but with a great deal of expertise, thanks to the fact that many of the officials have spent years working in the countries that are most likely to be affected.

But there have been tensions. Klaus Stohr, co-ordinator of WHO's global influenza programme, made an early prediction that there would be between 2 and 7 million deaths from a pandemic. This assessment was based on an extrapolation from the 1968 Hong Kong flu pandemic, which was a relatively mild pandemic although it still killed a million people worldwide. But a bombshell was dropped in September 2004 when that prediction suddenly leapt into stratospheric levels. Dr David Nabarro, newly appointed as the UN's most senior bird flu expert, said that the real number of deaths could be anything from 5 million to 150 million. His figures were swiftly rebutted by a WHO spokesman, but Dr Nabarro has made no apology for the high numbers.

A London-born scientist, seen by many as a highly political appointment in the WHO, Dr Nabarro has been banging the drum for much better co-ordination within national governments, because what worries him is that ministers often withhold information from one another as they fight over territory. 'I would like to see a person in each government given authority to bring all parts of government together for pandemic preparedness, and quickly,' he told *The Times* in October 2005. 'It is a job that could be done by the prime minister or deputy prime minister. The key to combating this threat is joined-up government. It was the same with SARS, and it will be the same with regards to influenza.'

The Western world's responsibility to poorer nations is an area he feels has been neglected. 'We need to get countries at the same level of preparedness for a pandemic so that they can contain and respond to the first clusters of human cases, and to the impact of a much wider distribution of human pandemic influenza. This is a global problem and reducing the risk in Britain and the US is not just a case of sorting yourselves out and getting your own supplies of Tamiflu.'

In November 2005, more than 600 delegates from over 100 countries met at a high-level WHO conference and agreed that there was urgent need for financial help for those nations already affected by bird flu. These are the key steps that experts believe have to be taken in response to the threat:

- Controlling the disease in birds at source, by improving veterinary services and through culling, vaccination and compensation schemes.

- Building up early detection and rapid response systems for H5N1.

- Making sure there are more laboratories to diagnose disease.

- Rapid containment of any animal or human clusters and training staff to investigate them.

- Testing national pandemic plans, holding a global emergency exercise and training more doctors to deal with bird flu.

- Helping countries to produce co-ordinated technical and financial support to see them through a pandemic.

- Ensuring that there is honest and factual communication with the public.

As Dr Lee Jong-Wook, head of WHO, commented at the end of the historic meeting: 'We have plans on paper, but we must now test them. Once a pandemic virus appears, it will be too late.'

From the many hours of discussion, what emerged seemed to be a new understanding between countries that they had to share their experiences and also their expertise in order to be able to combat the disease.

The World Bank's aim of raising $1 billion over the next three years to finance the investment in countries where the disease is endemic is ambitious but hugely important. The question now is whether the world's political leaders will still give the issue a high priority when it is no longer front-page news. The solutions – a good vaccine and proper surveillance measures – could take years to put in place.

One of the big breakthroughs in April 2005 was that the agriculture experts, virologists and veterinarians joined together through the auspices of the UN to create a new network of animal laboratories around the world, which could work together to share material, avoid duplication and decide which research areas to prioritize. A merger of the World Organization for Animal Health (also known as the OIE) and the UN's Food and Agriculture Organization (FAO), it has been given the unlikely but memorable acronym of OFFLU. Their plan is to work closely with the WHO so that more research can be done on the way that animal diseases move into human beings, and in particular to analyse more closely the current threat from avian flu.

7 BRITAIN'S RESPONSE TO THE THREAT

'I was always afraid of dying. Always. It was my fear that made me learn everything I could about my airplane and my emergency equipment, and kept me flying respectful of my machine and always alert in the cockpit.'

General Chuck Jeager — US fighter pilot, World War II

We are not fighting a war, yet at times the language used to discuss preparations for a flu pandemic can make it feel like an impending conflict. For a start, we are told about the need for 'resilience' among the public. There are emergency response teams being set up in every region, and exercises are being carried out to see how quickly they could react in a crisis. There are contingency plans to draft in the army to help distribute antiviral medications or to run the mortuaries, and the police may have to to deal with social unrest that could ensue during the initial panic. There is talk of curfews and quarantine, of shortages of drugs and closures of schools.

But Britain is not over-reacting. The government is doing exactly what the World Health Organization has asked each national government to do, which is to work out a plan for dealing with a flu pandemic that is as detailed as possible. The UK Influenza Pandemic Contingency Plan, first produced in March 2005 and then revised in October the same year, is an attempt to deal with as many of those uncertainties as possible.

It took the British government a while to wake up to the real threat of flu. In early 2004, when the first cases of human H5N1 infection appeared in Vietnam and Thailand, there was little interest in the matter. But by November that year, the Cabinet already had the issue of avian influenza on its agenda, and the then health secretary John Reid was under pressure to decide how much to spend on stockpiling anti-viral drugs.

' It remains unclear how patients who are sick will actually make it to the GP's surgery to get the medication they need.'

There are still gaping holes in our knowledge. We don't yet know, for example, which groups of workers would be prioritized either for vaccination or medication, given that guidelines will have to be set if the pandemic arrives before we have a full stockpile of drugs.

It remains unclear how patients who are sick will actually make it to the GP's surgery to get the medication they need. Will they be asked to go into voluntary quarantine instead and receive a home visit from health professionals? The way in which people receive medical help is a crucially important question that has to be fully answered by the government.

Many experts feel the UK is ahead of other nations when it comes to looking to the future. Sir Roy Anderson, chief adviser to the Ministry of Defence on infectious diseases, said he thought that we were 'better prepared than most' countries when it came to planning. That may be because Britain has lived through the BSE crisis and foot-and-mouth disease, both animal diseases which had an enormous impact on the country.

There is another crucial factor governing our ability to cope. The events of 11 September 2001 in the US and then the bombings of 7 July 2005 in London have spurred us on to create new ways of planning for emergencies. The lessons that were learned from those terrorist attacks have helped the police, ambulance services and others to work far more closely together to prepare for the unexpected. This chapter investigates how those plans are going – and where the gaps may lie.

THE MAN AT THE HELM

The man charged with preparing Britain for a flu pandemic has all the necessary qualifications, including one which is not on his CV – he has actually survived a flu pandemic himself, and remembers it well.

Back in 1968, when Sir Liam Donaldson was a medical student starting out on his career, he spent the summer studying at the renowned John Hopkins Medical School in Baltimore. While he was there, he decided he should visit his aunt who lived in New London, Connecticut. 'One evening, there was a great deal of coughing and spluttering going on around the dinner table and the next day I was completely laid low,' he recalled. 'I had to lie in bed in her house for seven or eight days with a high temperature, feeling delirious.' He recovered, and now as the country's chief medical officer he finds himself at the helm of this unprecedented effort to prepare the UK for another full-scale flu pandemic.

> *'"One evening, there was a great deal of coughing and spluttering going on around the dinner table and the next day I was completely laid low," he recalled.'*

Early in 2005, Sir Liam hit the headlines after telling journalists that it was a case of 'when, not if' a flu pandemic would come to our shores. In the last two months, he has been deluged with papers and documents assessing the risks, and pointing out what needs to be done.

Sir Liam, a man who prides himself on avoiding jargon and being as straightforward as possible, emphasizes that the pandemic threat is still exactly that – a threat – but he is deeply worried about the situation in Southeast Asia. The chances of containing the disease within one country when it emerges as a 'humanized' form are slim, he feels. 'I would be very surprised if we found out about human-to-human spread within 48 hours, quick enough to give the drugs,' he says. 'What is more likely to happen is that we will see multi-focal outbreaks [outbreaks in several places at once]. You still have to try to contain it, but I am pessimistic about the chances of doing so.'

Sir Liam hopes that when the virus looks as though it might be moving closer to a human pandemic strain, GPs will be given detailed guidance on the exact symptoms they should look for, because the disease will have its own 'signature', or pattern of illness. 'If it emerges in the Far East you could characterize the early symptoms and have a bit more specificity about what they look out for.' But he said that with medications that need to be given within 48 hours 'it is very dramatic, it is different to any other comparable situation or any other life-threatening emergency. We will have to invent a different way of getting the medicine to the patient as quickly as possible.'

'We will have to invent a different way of getting the medicine to the patient as quickly as possible.'

I asked him whether he was worried about the potential for hysteria and enormous social unrest created by such an emergency – and a shortage of Tamiflu.

'The other night, I was at a dinner at the Royal College of Physicians and one of the non-medical people tapped me on the shoulder and said, "I have a supply of Tamiflu, because I'm very worried about it. I have just developed a sore throat – do you think I should take it?" That's just what we don't want to happen,' he said.

'We need a bit of communitarism here. If we are unlucky and it comes before a full stockpile is in, we will have to be even tighter with the restrictions. I think people will realize that it wouldn't be fair if the store was depleted by people taking it if they just had a bit of a cold.

'My own feeling is that if you look at other things going on, we are quite an ordered country compared to some others. If you look at the bombings [London's terrorist bombings in July 2005], people did help others at risk to their own lives. How were they to know that there was not another bomb about to go off? What we have to do is to send the right message out to people – take responsibility not just for yourself and your family, but for your neighbours and others.'

THE SIX STAGES OF A PANDEMIC

In 2005, the World Health Organization revised its plan for dealing with the flu pandemic that might emerge at any time. This new six-stage plan is the basis on which each country has to prepare its own responses, both before, during and after the pandemic. It enables authorities to plan what they will need to do during each stage. At the time of going to press, we are in Phase 3 of this timetable. It will be Phase 5 that presents us with enormous uncertainty and fear, and within one to two months of the first large clusters of human cases being seen, we will find ourselves in Phase 6. You are likely to hear far more about these different stages in the months to come as the virus evolves and changes. The six phases leading to a pandemic, according to the WHO plan, revised in 2005 are:

- **Phase 1.** No new influenza virus subtypes have been found in humans. If one is present in animals, risk of human disease is low.

- **Phase 2.** A circulating animal influenza virus poses a substantial risk of human disease.

- **Phase 3.** Human infections with a new subtype, but no new human-to-human spread.

- **Phase 4.** Small clusters with limited human-to-human spread but virus still not well adapted to people.

- **Phase 5.** Large clusters, virus becoming better adapted to people, but not yet fully transmissible.

- **Phase 6.** Pandemic phase. Virus is spreading right across the general population.

HOW TO GET MEDICAL TREATMENT IN THE EVENT OF A PANDEMIC

The number of people in the UK likely to be infected by pandemic flu is estimated at around 14 million, representing 25 per cent of the population. That is an enormous number but it is worth keeping in mind that the large majority will suffer nothing more than a nasty bout of flu. However, a substantial minority is likely to develop complications. The real difficulty for the NHS would be how to care for those patients who develop breathing difficulties, pneumonia or bronchitis. The complication rate could be as high as 10 per cent of those infected, which in the UK would amount to 1.4 million people.

'The number of people in the UK likely to be infected by pandemic flu is estimated at around 14 million, representing 25 per cent of the population.'

What should people do when they first develop symptoms? There are several options that are still being considered by the Department of Health. The first line of treatment will be the anti-viral medication oseltamivir, or Tamiflu, which really needs to be taken within 48 hours of the first symptoms appearing. When the doctors say 'symptoms', what they mean is a collection of different signs of illness that will be particular to pandemic flu. This may be a high temperature and coughing, or it could be aching muscles and a headache. One of the problems with flu is that the symptoms can be quite varied, but in the case of a pandemic strain there may be a recognizable pattern of illness.

How will people get the drug? There will probably be four or five options open to them.

The first will be to go to a GP's surgery and wait to see a doctor. However, sitting in a doctor's waiting room when you feel very ill is not a good idea. Patients are at the peak of the infectious period in the first two days, so it would be better for them to stay away. Currently the drug can only be prescribed by a doctor, but that rule may be relaxed during a pandemic.

The second option being considered by the government is for anyone who is sick with flu to receive a home visit. Sir Liam wants to see if nurses or other healthcare staff could be trained to go into homes, check patients' temperatures and assess their symptoms, and then advise them what to do. These home visitors may be able to dispense drugs without recourse to a doctor. This could turn out to be the most practical option. The Royal College of Nursing is keen to see its profession help should it be needed but they realize that as many nurses would also catch flu themselves, they may need to ask retired nurses to help. They are also considering training extra staff to meet the possible demand and alleviate pressure on doctors.

The third option is to go to the casualty department at the local hospital, but the problem again is that patients might be infecting others and they could have a long wait before they were able to see a doctor. For the majority of patients, a hospital bed won't be needed, so they would just get some Tamiflu and be sent home for bedrest.

The fourth option is that pharmacists may be able to dispense the drug without a doctor's prescription, but there are fears that they would not be able to cope with the demand.

> *'Those running NHS Direct are already looking at how you would 'triage' patients by asking them to describe their symptoms in detail, so they can diagnose and prioritize the most needy.'*

Another possibility is that in order to receive help in the first place, patients would have to contact NHS Direct. This is a telephone helpline service run by the NHS that takes thousands of calls each year, but which might come into its own during a pandemic. Those running NHS Direct are already looking at how you would 'triage' patients by asking them to describe their symptoms in detail, so they can diagnose and prioritize the most needy. The operators could then give callers advice on whether they needed to see a nurse or doctor, or the easiest way for them to obtain a supply of Tamiflu in their area.

THE PRESSURE ON INTENSIVE CARE UNITS

Those who develop complications may need to be given antibiotics or hospitalized. If many hundreds of thousands of people became seriously ill, no health service would be able to offer each of them a ventilator and full emergency support. The demand for a bed could rise to far beyond anything the hospitals could currently offer. Roughly 7 per cent of those who fall ill may need a ventilator, a machine that assists your breathing when your lungs are in trouble, and the NHS does not remotely have enough to help everyone.

It might be necessary to come up with some different solutions and ways of offering care at the height of a pandemic. The Intensive Care Society, an organization of doctors who run intensive care units across Britain, is looking at plans that would see all elective, non-urgent hospital work cancelled, so that thousands of beds could be used for the most severe cases of flu. They are also checking their stocks of vital equipment, such as ventilators and syringe infusion pumps, which are used to pump drugs such as antibiotics into the patients.

'Roughly 7 per cent of those who fall ill may need a ventilator, a machine that assists your breathing when your lungs are in trouble, and the NHS does not remotely have enough to help everyone.'

Dr David Menon, professor of anaesthetics at Addenbrooke's Hospital in Cambridge and a member of the Intensive Care Society's council, told me that a flu pandemic would put an enormous burden on intensive care, so that they had to look at new ways of dealing with so many sick. 'The number of ITU patients needing ventilation might rise by over 230 per cent during a three-month pandemic period, so to deal with that you would have to double our capacity, which would be impossible. Instead we have to look at other parts of a hospital which could be used. But the staffing is also crucial, and some staff will also be off sick with the flu, so we have to make allowances for that.'

THE WAIT FOR A VACCINATION PROGRAMME

More than 120 million doses of vaccine have been ordered by the government to protect people against H5N1 when it eventually mutates into a human strain. This is enough for two doses per

How many would be affected?

The figures below indicate the scale of the challenge that would confront the health service if a relatively mild virus hit a town the size of Dover, with a population of 104,000, in a pandemic that lasted for three months.

- *25,000 people would be infected with pandemic flu*
- *2,500 of these would need a consultation with their GP*
- *1,250 patients would go to accident and emergency for help*
- *140 patients would become seriously ill with acute respiratory problems*
- *90 people would die as a result of the virus.*

person, because the research so far suggests that this will be the amount needed. (See pages 98–103 for more about vaccines.)

In October 2005, Sir Liam Donaldson announced that the UK would take out 'sleeping contracts' with vaccine manufacturers, so that they could start to prepare for a pandemic. Putting in an early order for a product that hasn't yet been made gives the pharmaceutical companies a chance to expand their capacity – both workforce and factories – before an outbreak, and it also means that Britain will be at the front of the queue for the vaccine.

But there is a hitch. The vaccine cannot be manufactured until the virus has actually mutated into a strain which spreads easily between people, because until then its genetic make-up won't be known. Without that detail, the vaccine might not be accurate enough to create the correct immune response. The eventual immunization programme won't be ready until between four and six months after the flu first becomes 'humanized'. That means that it might not be available until the pandemic is well underway. However, it could still be used to deal with successive waves of infection or given to people who had managed to avoid infection up to that point.

Sir Liam told a packed press conference at the Department of Health in October 2005: 'We cannot prevent a flu pandemic, but we can reduce its impact. We will use this vaccine to immunize the UK population, and reduce the impact of a pandemic on society.'

How safe would a vaccine be? No one can answer that yet but the vaccine, even though it was being rushed out for a pandemic which could kill millions, would still have to go through safety trials to prove it did not cause harmful side effects. There would have to be careful consideration of what kind of dose children might need, or whether pregnant women could be vaccinated.

Britain has also ordered two million doses of an early vaccine that works against the current strain of H5N1. It won't be a perfect immunisation by any means, because the virus will have changed by the time it becomes a pandemic, but this small stockpile is an insurance policy, because it could offer some limited protection to healthcare workers, before the proper vaccine is made.

'There would have to be careful consideration of what kind of dose children might need, or whether pregnant women could be vaccinated.'

CLOSING DOWN BRITAIN

Experts fear that if the disease becomes contagious between people, someone boarding a plane in a place like Hong Kong could spread the virus around the world in a matter of hours. 'You'd be surprised how fast that virus can travel from a Third World, backward country farm into New York City,' said Dr Frederick Leung of Hong Kong University, who has studied the avian virus for years. 'I bet it is faster than a terrorist can arrive. Of course, viruses observe no country boundaries. The virus doesn't apply for a visa to go travel.'

Closing all the airports may feel like the right action to take, but the truth is that it would ultimately be ineffective against a virus which is so easily transmissible between people. The UK's Contingency Plan makes it clear that the disease may be unstoppable once a new influenza virus capable of causing serious illness appears. It states bluntly that 'even a 99.9 per cent restriction of travel into the country would only be expected to delay importation of the virus by up to two months.'

The plan adds, 'Spread from the source country to the UK, through the movement of people, is likely to take around a month, and experience of the dissemination of SARS from Hong Kong suggests modern travel may result in wide international spread even more rapidly than this.' Officials have seen data which suggests that an outbreak starting in Hong Kong would take between two and four weeks to reach London.

Airline companies have already been told by the UK's Department of Transport not to carry sick passengers, particularly those coming from Southeast Asia. They have the legal right to turn away anyone who appears unwell. But the virus takes 24 hours to incubate so it is possible that someone could board a flight seeming fine and then subsequently become very ill.

By 2006, posters will be going up in airports around the UK to warn passengers that if they feel unwell they should not be getting on a flight. The port authorities have also asked their staff to look out for travellers who appear to be sick on arrival in the UK.

'Airline companies have already been told by the UK's Department of Transport not to carry sick passengers, particularly those coming from Southeast Asia.'

Given that closing the borders will delay but not prevent the virus from arriving, should all the airports and ports be closed if the virus reaches Europe? There is an argument that it might win us some precious time to prepare for the emergency, but politicians have been told that it could just end up harming the economy for longer than necessary. At the moment, there are no travel restrictions in place, but people who have come from infected countries such as Romania and Turkey are subject to entry checks at Heathrow and Gatwick, with sniffer dogs checking that they are not bringing in any food products, especially birds or eggs.

Each region of Britain now has its own regional 'resilience committee', a group made up of police officers, ambulance staff, health experts and local authority representatives who are there to look at all possible needs that might arise from different kinds of disasters. Clearly, the plan for dealing with a pandemic lasting three months or more will be different from the kind of plan they devise to deal with the local river flooding – but the services that you would rely on remain the same. It is interesting that in the capital, the London Regional Resilience Forum has learned lessons from the 7 July bombings that are now feeding into their plans for dealing with a flu pandemic. One of those, for example, is that in an emergency, you can't necessarily rely on mobile phones. When the bombs went off on 7 July, some emergency staff couldn't communicate with each other because the mobile networks went down. In a pandemic, effective telecommunications would have to be safeguarded. Similarly, the police discovered that when they went on TV after the bombings to ask the public to avoid using the 999 service until they knew the full situation, the public responded very well. The same message might be necessary again at the full height of a pandemic.

'When the bombs went off on 7 July, some emergency staff couldn't communicate with each other because the mobile networks went down.'

Planners in each area also have to look at business continuity planning and transport measures, to try and limit the damage to the economy. Some of the duties they might have to fulfill are described in the remainder of this chapter.

WOULD QUARANTINE BE ENFORCED?

Ever since the Black Death swept across Europe in the 14th century, successive ages have resorted to quarantine in an attempt to stop the spread of infectious diseases. But whether the practice of isolating people from one another has ever worked very well is highly debatable, according to medical historians.

The term 'quarantine' comes from the Italian phrase *quaranta giorni* (forty days), signifying the length of time ships were kept isolated before they were allowed to enter the port of Dubrovnik in the Middle Ages, as a way of keeping out the Black Death. In 1490, quarantines were enforced around Europe to check the spread of syphilis infections, and in the early 19th cen-

Travel advice

What about those who want to travel to Southeast Asia or other infected regions? So far, the news about bird flu doesn't appear to have made a dent in the tourist trade to these countries.

Dr Richard Dawood, a specialist at the Fleet Street Travel Clinic in London, advises that travellers should not be put off visiting the region, but that they should avoid any contact with birds, especially at large 'wet markets' where live birds are traded.

'There is absolutely no risk at present for anyone wishing to travel to Southeast Asia,' he said. 'The number of humans who have caught the infection from birds have been directly in contact with them, and it is a tiny number compared with the number of birds carrying the disease.'

Backpackers are at no more risk than business travellers, according to Dr Dawood, but it is still sensible to avoid contact with live birds if possible. He does think that it is a good idea to have the jab for normal winter flu before travelling, because if there were a sudden outbreak of the virus, someone with normal flu symptoms might find themselves put into quarantine – as they were during the SARS crisis. 'Unfortunately, we are rapidly running out of the [normal] flu vaccine,' said Dr Dawood. 'Because of heightened concerns, many more people than usual have come forward for immunization this winter.'

---

tury it was used to try and prevent the entry of yellow fever into Spain, but they did nothing to stop the spread of the disease. Quarantine was also used during the SARS epidemic in 2003 (see page 175). Now, with the threat of a flu pandemic, people are talking again about how quarantine might work, but there are many ethical issues to be discussed.

The government still needs to answer a number of questions.

Would quarantine be voluntary or would it be enforced? If it was compulsory for a family who had been exposed to a flu case, who would enforce it? And how long would people be expected to remain under quarantine?

The British contingency plan talks about 'social distancing measures' that might need to be taken in the event of a pandemic, but falls short of explaining how they would work. The general consensus seems to be that when the pandemic virus first arrives in Britain, putting people who have been exposed to it into quarantine might work for a few weeks but ultimately it would not halt the spread of the disease, and would probably not affect the number of people who became infected.

'Would quarantine be voluntary or would it be enforced? If it was compulsory for a family who had been exposed to a flu case, who would enforce it?'

Those who have been exposed to the flu may be asked to stay at home to prevent them spreading it – and if they refuse to comply, the police could be asked to enforce quarantine. But this is a step which officials are loathe to take. Compulsory quarantine would only work in the initial four to six weeks of the pandemic, because after that the disease would be very widespread, and it would be impossible for the police to impose it on so many.

Closing schools is also a difficult issue. The government has not yet made a decision about whether education authorities would be instructed to close schools in the event of a local outbreak. Although such a move might initially reduce the spread of the disease among children, it probably wouldn't ultimately affect the number of infected cases, because families would still come into contact with others during the expected three- to four-month period a pandemic might last.

The plan also states: 'Closing schools will have an impact on maintaining the workforce in other sectors.' In other words, when schools close, it is often women who would stay at home to look after the children, and that might have a very damaging impact on the economy.

Sir Liam Donaldson is trying to keep all the options open for as long as possible when it comes to social measures. 'I don't think you can be rigid about this,' he told me. 'You have to try and respond to the circumstances in which you find yourself. For example, if pandemic flu arrived in Southend, and there was an outbreak limited to a small community, you might want to close schools in the area to limit movement initially. But this is a disease that will spread everywhere, so you can't build all your plans around it.'

THE ROLE OF THE POLICE

There's a strong possibility of widespread social unrest during a flu pandemic, particularly as demand for anti-viral medications will be sky-high but there will be no easy access to them. Police guards might have to be placed on doctors' surgeries and NHS clinics in the event of a pandemic to control patients who might become unreasonable and start demanding the anti-viral drugs. These suggestions

'Police guards might have to be placed on doctors' surgeries and NHS clinics in the event of a pandemic to control patients who might become unreasonable and start demanding the anti-viral drugs.'

are outlined in a report drawn up by a senior planner for the Metropolitan Police Authority in London, which was submitted to the House of Lords Science and Technology Committee in November 2005 when it held an inquiry into Britain's plans for a flu pandemic. Other forces throughout the United Kingdom have also been instructed to prepare for the possibility of a pandemic in the next few years.

Giving evidence to the committee, Alan Goodwin, Deputy Chief Constable of Derbyshire Constabulary and chair of the emergency planning committee for the Association of Chief Police Officers, said that providing information to the public about what was happening would be essential. He told the committee: 'For me, a key part of that communication strategy would be: do our staff, do our 999 call-takers, do our call centre call-takers actually have the information to hand to give people who are ringing in – possibly in a distressed or panicked state – to be able to satisfy that query?' At the same time, he said, the local police officer in the street would have to be able to offer reassurance. But he made it clear that a pandemic would put them (and any other service) under huge pressure because they themselves would have staff off sick.

Alan Goodwin said that they would have to try to maintain a core service to the public at the same time as responding to the pandemic situation. 'There is certainly the potential for military assistance if that is required. If it were a sporadic outbreak in terms of geographical location, there are the facilities to be able to call upon police resources from other parts of the country that perhaps have not been affected in that way.'

'It is likely that large public events such as football matches and concerts would be cancelled in order to prevent spread of disease.'

It is likely that large public events such as football matches and concerts would be cancelled in order to prevent spread of disease. Medium-sized gatherings, however, of fewer than 50 people, may be allowed – although whether anyone would go to them in the middle of such an emergency is another matter.

PREPARING FOR MASS FATALITIES

The UK, like all other countries, has been asked by the World Health Organization to calculate a range of possible mortality rates in the event of a pandemic. This is based on various estimates of how many people might be infected and the lethality of the virus.

Experts have calculated that if the disease has a 'clinical attack rate' of 25 per cent – i.e. it infects that percentage of the UK population – and 1 per cent of those people die, then there would be 141,000 deaths. But if the virus proves more lethal and its 'overall case fatality rate' rises to 1.5 per cent, then the number of deaths would rise to 212,000. If it has the same fatality rate as was seen in the 1918 pandemic (2.5 per cent), the number of dead would increase to a staggering 355,000.

If it was like the 1957 pandemic, the fatality rate could be as low as 0.37 per cent, which would mean 53,700 deaths. But really, as the government's pandemic plan says, this figure 'has been used to illustrate the minimum that might be expected, even with treatment.'

What could planners do when faced with such massive numbers of deaths? Within government, it is the Civil Contingencies Secretariat that has to provide local and regional authorities with the information they need to respond to civil emergencies. One of the areas the local committees have to consider is preparation for mass fatalities. There is already a team of experts working on a 'mass mortality plan' for London, for example.

Planners have been asked to identify areas within each district that could operate as makeshift mortuaries if the local facilities were unable to cope. They have also had to work out where the manpower would come from to run the mortuaries, and to help remove bodies from homes if the pandemic was overwhelming the undertakers.

Local coroners might have to change the rules about ordering post mortems on people who have died at home unsupervised by healthcare workers. It might also be necessary to tell bereaved families that their loved ones can't be buried, but have to be cremated instead. This is not because the corpses would spread infection, but because of the sheer numbers needing interment, for which there might not be space in existing graveyards.

EFFECTS ON FARMING AND THE COUNTRYSIDE

There's a horrible sense of déjà vu about the threat of disease getting into poultry. During the foot-and-mouth outbreak of 2001, Britain saw its countryside effectively closed down amid fear that tourists and walkers could unwittingly spread the disease. TV images of cattle being herded towards the sheds for culling, surrounded by men in white boiler suits and masks, were shocking. The crisis cost the UK some £4 billion, and led to the slaughter of more than 6 million animals.

If bird flu comes to Britain and infects any of our poultry flocks, it is likely that all poultry will be ordered indoors. This has already happened in most parts of France and some of Germany, as well as all of the Netherlands. As some 25 per cent of British flocks are now free-range, it will impose an enormous cost burden on farmers who will have to build proper indoor facilities. Some will not be able to do so, and it is likely that many thousands of chickens would be culled, either by gassing or by being electrically stunned.

Isolation zones would be set up around the afflicted farms, but it is highly unlikely that entire communities would be cut off. Nearby villages might face extra security measures, however, such as disinfecting farm equipment and even car tyres as they drove in and out of the area. There could also be an immediate ban on Britain exporting poultry to the rest of the EU until flocks had been given the all-clear.

One lesson that was learned during foot-and-mouth disease was that it was mostly spread by the rapid and uncontrolled movements of livestock around the country. Poultry owners may be faced with enormous restrictions on movement of birds until vets have verified they are disease-free. They will also have to make sure their workers are well protected with proper masks, gloves and suits.

The big fear for the food and farming industry is that because of bird flu, consumers will turn away from eating poultry and eggs. For this reason, the government has already tried to reassure the public that it is safe to eat both, provided that they are properly cooked – although industry bosses feel they haven't been reassuring enough.

In evidence presented to a House of Lords select committee in November 2005, it emerged that the sales of chicken had fallen by between 5 and 10 per cent since the issue of bird flu hit the UK headlines the previous month.

Kevin Hawkins, director-general of the British Retail Consortium, was quietly scathing about the government's response when asked about it by the Lords committee. Apparently angered by the fact that in a TV appearance Sir Liam Donaldson had just talked in 'medical terms' about bird flu, he accused government departments of not co-ordinating their messages and doing enough to reassure the public over the safety of chicken.

'What has become clear to date is that there does not seem to be a great deal of co-ordination between government departments, particularly the Department of Health and Defra and, of course, the Food Standards Agency,' he told them when he gave evidence on 3 November. 'We saw this again during foot and mouth, and it seems to be the case now that the government does not really get its act together and speak with one voice at the same time.'

During a pandemic of human flu, the concerns about food would change from issues of safety to issues of availability. How would food reach us during a pandemic? The directors of the big supermarket chains have all been called in to meetings with the government, and asked to prepare plans to ensure that vital supplies would still make it through to their major stores. All the big supermarkets are currently looking at how their key goods – including milk, bread, baby food, toilet rolls and disinfectant – might reach consumers, how much might be needed and what would happen if some smaller stores were closed. As many of their staff are women, who are likely to want to stay at home with their children during a flu crisis, they face particular staffing problems.

'...it emerged that the sales of chicken had fallen by between 5 and 10 per cent since the issue of bird flu hit the UK headlines the previous month.'

The main point of vulnerability in the food supply chain, according to Kevin Hawkins, would be the heavy goods vehicle drivers – the people who get the food from manufacturers to the retail distribution centres run by supermarkets. There is already a shortage of qualified HGV drivers and if even 10 per cent of them fell sick at the same time, they could not be replaced.

'The other problem, of course, would be panic buying,' Mr Hawkins told the committee. 'When people believe that by going out of doors and going into food stores they are increasing the risk of them catching some disease, then they would tend to panic buy to hoard and to keep indoors for as long as the crisis lasted. We would have to move very quickly to ensure that there was no panic buying.'

COULD HOUSEHOLD PETS CATCH BIRD FLU?

If a pandemic came to Britain, would cats, dogs, rabbits, guinea pigs and other pets catch the virus? Given that H5N1 has already shown a propensity to infect other species – including tigers, leopards, pigs and cats – it's not impossible that our domesticated animals would suffer.

Studies have shown that domestic cats can be infected with the H5N1 virus, and that they can pass it on to other cats. What is not known is whether they could then pass the disease on to humans. Cats don't shed the virus in the same way that birds and poultry do, so even if they caught flu, it may not be as contagious for their owners. Dogs, on the other hand, appear so far to have escaped the virus in Southeast Asia. And vets have said that there is very little risk of pet birds catching bird flu.

'No one currently knows whether pets could catch the virus from humans, or whether they could act as carriers, passing it on to people or other species.'

No one currently knows whether pets could catch the virus from humans, or whether they could act as carriers, passing it on to people or other species. Until the virus mutates and becomes a human form, it's impossible to predict exactly how it might spread into other species. For the government, therefore, it is impossible to formulate any kind of advice for pet owners on what to do until they know the extent of the threat facing domestic animals.

The RSPCA believe there is very little chance of pet dogs or cats catching bird flu from birds. 'While it is possible a cat or dog could become infected with the virus, unless there is significant exposure and a weak immune system, the risk to pets is very small.'

However, the Hong Kong government has taken a more cautious approach, advising the public not to kiss their pets. According to the Hong Kong Agriculture, Fisheries and Conservation Department, owners should wash their hands after touching birds, wear gloves while cleaning up droppings and always keep pets away from human food. These are precautions that sensible pet owners would take anyway.

WHAT WOULD HAPPEN TO BRITISH INDUSTRY?

The risks for any company trying to carry on business as normal during a flu pandemic are enormous. Unlike an act of terrorism, a hurricane or a flood, this will not be a dire, one-off event leaving people without office buildings or computer equipment. The major impact will be caused by staff being too sick, or deciding not to come to work, for the duration of the outbreak, which could be three months or more.

The government predicts that normal sickness rates of between 2 and 6 per cent of the workforce would be likely to double in the case of a pandemic, and that up to 25 per cent of workers would be absent for between five and eight days over a three-month period. However, that could be a huge underestimate. Some companies are working on the basis that you might have as much as 60 per cent of your workforce off at any one time. This represents a massive shortfall in employees, both for larger and smaller companies.

Research by the Chartered Management Institute in the UK shows that despite these risks, most businesses have given little consideration to the possible impact of a flu pandemic. Business continuity plans – the strategies for dealing with such crises – tend to concentrate not on staff, but on the other more tangible risks, such as loss of IT capacity, loss of telecommunications, fire, inability to get on the site, or terrorist damage.

Hugh Leighton, of the risk consultancy company Aon Limited, commented recently, 'Businesses must acknowledge that the outbreak of a flu pandemic is a genuine risk and one of the greatest threats to future performance. Experts describe an outbreak in terms of "when", not "if".

The UK pandemic plan asks companies to consider all the following criteria, no matter how difficult it might seem at first:

• Establishing minimum staffing levels

• Identifying a 'front line' group of essential staff

• Considering whether some staff could be redeployed to do jobs they might not be trained to do

• Considering recruiting additional staff or volunteers

• Accommodation such as portacabins with bunk beds for people to rest in between shifts, in case transport home is disrupted

• The amount of leave staff might need to ensure they could carry on working at increased levels over several weeks.

'Unlike fire or flooding, a flu pandemic would be an uninsured event and the cost of it would have to be absorbed by the business.'

One of the big differences that has occurred in industry between the 1968 pandemic and the present day is the globalization of trade. Many UK companies use overseas suppliers and have integrated 'just in time' techniques, which are based on goods reaching them with very little delay. Clearly, if an outbreak begins in the Far East, with its enormous manufacturing base, there is a huge risk to the supply chain. If materials are quarantined as a result of a pandemic, then there would be a direct hit to profits.

Unlike fire or flooding, a flu pandemic would be an uninsured event and the cost of it would have to be absorbed by the business. That is why experts are calling for chairmen and directors to make it a top priority. 'To ignore this risk is tantamount to a dereliction of duty,' said Hugh Leighton. 'We encourage all companies to assess their current level of preparedness and to take measures to mitigate against the disruption caused by a potential outbreak. Every day that a pandemic is delayed is another day for business leaders to prepare. Business continuity planning is the first and only line of defence.'

Computers would come into their own during a pandemic

Preparing for the worst

Bob Piggott does not think of himself as a natural pessimist. But as head of group risk management for the banking giant HSBC, it is only right that he considers the worst scenarios when looking at the future. With 245,000 employees in 79 different countries, HSBC has had to formulate a strategy that will help everyone, although it can be adapted for different national needs.

He is amazed that companies worldwide are not doing more to prepare for the natural disaster which he believes is on its way, sooner or later. 'We suffered with SARS – we lost an employee in Hong Kong to the disease. But with that infection at least you could quarantine people against it. The same won't be true of pandemic flu, and we have to accept that.'

His plan is about as well advanced as it is possible to be, given the enormous uncertainties around how, and when the virus will mutate into a human form. 'In Britain, we have 45,000 staff, the vast majority of them working in the branches, and they are not in a position to work using remote access from home. Many of our staff are women, and they may have to care for children if the schools close, or care for other relatives. We are working on the basis that 60 per cent of staff will be off at any one point during the pandemic. The question is, how do we keep things running over a three-month period?'

The bank is looking at a number of options. This includes flexible working hours, so people could avoid travelling on public transport during rush hour, for example. It would also expand call centres' capability so that more people could pay bills by phone, instead of needing to come into a branch. They are preparing information for staff on hygiene in the home and in the workplace, as a measure which could cut infection rates.

(continued over)

However, within his sector there are big worries about money supply. 'Cash is very important. It's one of the few commodities that you will have to have in such a crisis, and we have to look at how we will keep the ATMs stocked up and running.'

He feels that the government has not done enough to make companies aware of the enormous challenges faced by pandemic flu — and the fact that they need to get moving with their plans. 'I managed to get it on the agenda of our last board meeting, with the chairman's support, because it is understood here now that this is serious,' he said. 'Given how fast this flu is going to spread between countries, I'd hope that we could react sooner, rather than later.'

situation, because many workers would want to stay at home, either through fear or because they are caring for someone who is ill. Businesses have been told that they need to step up their IT planning for a flu pandemic, to help people who can't get into the office.

The Confederation of British Industry (CBI) and the Institute of Directors have advised firms to do more to allow remote access to IT systems, and they also want to find out how many companies would be able to communicate electronically with customers and suppliers if transport was disrupted or offices had to be quarantined.

HOW THE PUBLIC WILL BE KEPT IN THE PICTURE

Warning people what to expect and how to behave during an emergency is vital if we are to avoid panic. The term 'public information campaign' has a 1950s ring to it. People are not that keen on them because they have the ring of a 'nanny state' about them, but when there is a big emergency these messages become crucially important.

Campaigns do more than give practical advice. They also serve the purpose of reassuring a jumpy populace that something is being done to deal with the problem. Far from panicking people, they usually attempt to calm things down, while at the same time giving some clear, practical steps to take.

The government is preparing to dust off a big TV and advertising radio campaign that it had prepared for the SARS crisis in 2003, but never actually used. Many of those messages still hold true, especially about the way in which you can cut down on the spread of germs.

During the 1957 pandemic, there was a catchy public health message: 'Coughs and sneezes spread diseases. Catch your germs in a handkerchief.' This was broadcast over the radio and also appeared on posters all over the cities, adorned with a picture of a boy sneezing into a hankie.

As the government's pandemic plan states: 'Communications are a crucial element of the response. Many groups, not least the public, will need clear, accurate information and advice about the actions they can take. They will also need assurance that their concerns are being addressed.'

'People do take these messages on board, provided they follow what I call the three Cs,' said Ron Finlay, Chief Executive of the media consultancy group Fishburn Hedges. 'There has to be Credibility, Consultation and Consistency. Firstly, the information in the messages has to be accurate and comprehensive. Secondly, the government would have to consult with the medical community and other groups to make sure everyone knew what was happening, and lastly, there has to be consistency between those messages and what other people say. If you get entirely different advice coming, say, from another group of health professionals, that could be really damaging.'

The likely sequence of public communications, as outlined in the government's pandemic plan, will be as follows:

• At Phase 4 (when there are small clusters of flu with limited human-to-human spread): A leaflet explaining the key facts and giving practical self-help advice will drop through every letterbox in the country. It will also be available on the Department of Health's website (see page 216). A public information film will be broadcast on the BBC and ITV explaining what pandemic flu is, and how it differs from the normal kind.

- At Phase 5 (when there are larger clusters of flu with more human-to-human spread): A big advertising campaign will begin, based on the previous campaign about SARS infections. As the pandemic plan states, 'The role of this advertising will be to alert the public that pandemic flu is almost certain to arrive in the UK imminently.' It will explain the difficulties faced in making a vaccine available, while at the same time emphasizing that work to develop one is ongoing. Lastly, it will talk about the importance of hygiene measures and infection control (see Chapter 8).

- At Phase 6 (when the virus is spreading across the general population): On the day that the UK enters a pandemic period (in other words, when human-to-human flu arrives here), Sir Liam Donaldson will address the nation, talking directly to camera about what the nation must do. It will be akin to Churchill's wartime radio messages, minus the cigar. There will then be rolling TV ads, and press conferences to update the media on the latest developments.

In the meantime, no one should panic. Humanized bird flu is more likely than not to reach Britain, but it may not be as devastating as some experts think. As Professor Colin Blakemore, chief executive of Britain's Medical Research Council, says, 'Vigilance and attention without panic is what we need at the moment.'

8 HOW TO PREPARE FOR A PANDEMIC

'Your general state of health may have some bearing on how you fare but it is dwarfed, in terms of risk, by whether or not you are exposed to the virus.'

Dr John Watson — Health Protection Agency

A raging fever, a headache and a cough that leaves you feeling exhausted: these may be the first signs of pandemic flu, although the illness will probably have its own pattern of symptoms when it becomes a fully human strain. For the vast majority of people, the illness they suffer will be no worse than a very nasty bout of flu. Sufferers will take to their beds feeling feverish and exhausted, and at times even light-headed and delirious. For some, however, the sickness will be far more serious and there will be complications that could prove fatal. At the time of writing, there is simply no way of knowing exactly how lethal this virus would be or which age group would be most vulnerable.

Given everything that has been said and written about bird flu to date, it's very easy to shrug your shoulders and think that there is nothing you can do about it. The prospect of an outbreak sweeping across Britain within weeks and claiming thousands of lives seems like an unstoppable act of fate against which we would all be powerless. There won't be any instant cure for a pandemic flu strain, that's for sure. As I explained in Chapter 5, a vaccine will take between four and six months to prepare, and scientists are already warning that Tamiflu is not a wonder drug.

But it is extremely important for people to know that they are not impotent against the threat. There are some simple, inexpensive and commonsense steps you can take that will leave you in a much better position to cope with the events before, during and after a flu pandemic. Some of the steps I outline in this chapter follow straightforward government advice; others are measures which have been adopted in other countries or recommended by experts, but which you won't find in the UK's official hand-out.

At a time of high anxiety, there are always dozens of health quacks making extraordinary claims about new cures for this, that and the next thing, and there are bound to be plenty of them about when it comes to bird flu. In this chapter, I don't recommend anything that is risky or for which there is no good evidence based on sound research and testing. Instead, I have outlined a broad approach that will help everyone, particularly families, to face the challenge of bird flu.

THE ROLE OF THE IMMUNE SYSTEM

It's very tempting to think that you could fend off pandemic flu by boosting the immune system in some way, with vitamins, exercise or special therapies. Some products do seem to help us in fighting off other viruses; echinacea, for example, appears to help us resist the common cold. But however attractive this idea sounds, it's not going to work with pandemic flu. Unlike the common cold, the immune system won't be able to recognize the attacker because it will be a completely new strain of virus (see Chapter 1). And the unpalatable truth is that with a pandemic strain of flu, it may be that a healthy immune system can act too vigorously in a way that harms rather than defends you.

One reason for the very high mortality rate among 20- to 40-year-olds during the 1918 pandemic was that they had too strong an immune response and in the body's attempt to fight off the viral invader it ended up destroying its own tissue. Here's what can happen. When your body is under attack, small, specialized proteins known as cytokines activate the B- and T-lymphocytes in white blood cells to repel the virus. If it's a totally foreign and unrecognizable virus, however, they won't be able to fight it off. Instead, they go into attack mode and provoke a strong inflammatory response in the lung tissue, known as a 'cytokine storm'. The tissue starts to break down and fluid and blood begin to leak out into the lungs. Before doctors can stop it, the lungs are filling up with liquid. This is what scientists are seeing when they look at the x-rays of patients in Vietnam who succumbed to H5N1. Many of them didn't die of secondary infections, such as pneumonia, but of their own inflammatory response.

'And the unpalatable truth is that with a pandemic strain of flu, it may be that a healthy immune system can act too vigorously in a way that harms rather than defends you.'

A study published in November 2005 in the journal *Respiratory Research* revealed that in human cells the H5N1 virus can trigger levels of inflammatory proteins more than ten times higher than the common human flu virus H1N1.

Despite this rather grim warning, it seems likely that someone in good general health would recover from flu more rapidly, with fewer complications, than someone who is malnourished or in bad health. The healthier you are, the more successfully your organs, such as heart, liver and lungs, will be able to withstand the virus. Research has consistently shown that a good diet, regular activity, lack of stress and plenty of sleep all play an important role in our ability to fight off disease.

Dr Adam Carey, nutritionist with the English Rugby Union, has written a lot about balanced diets and told me: 'I think that people should think about better nutrition rather than taking more vitamins. Unfortunately, there isn't that much hard evidence to show that taking extra vitamin C even fends off the common cold, so I can't see how it would work on pandemic flu.

'If people could eat a balanced diet, high in fresh products with lots of veg and fruit that are in season, rather than relying on highly processed food, that would benefit the entire body and its organs. We know that people who have poor nutrition, who live on a diet of junk, really struggle when it comes to fighting off infections. The liver in particular is really badly affected.'

Dr Carey says that taking a multivitamin pill wouldn't do any harm, but there isn't any evidence that it would help against a very virulent strain of flu. 'My view is that if you begin to eat well now, you'd face a flu outbreak in a much better state of health. It might not stop you being infected, but it might help you deal with complications of flu.'

'We know that people who have poor nutrition, who live on a diet of junk, really struggle when it comes to fighting off infections. The liver in particular is really badly affected.'

Of all the possible therapies and supplements that you could take during a pandemic, he singled out Omega-3 as the one that might really help. 'We generally have a lack of essential fatty acids in our diet, and Omega 3 is important. Given that in an emergency situation, you might find it hard to buy oily fish, it wouldn't be unreasonable to take this supplement. These essential fatty acids make prostaglandins which have an anti-inflammatory activity so they may help immune function.'

Any dietary improvements should be started several months before a potential pandemic to ensure you are in the best possible position to withstand the virus. And the same is certainly true of my next piece of advice…

GIVE UP SMOKING!

Do it now! Don't wait for another reason, or until it looks as if bird flu has become a humanized disease and has reached the shores of Britain. It is your lung cells which will take the burden of this virus if you become infected, and the healthier your lungs are generally, the less prone they will be to influenza and the complications it can bring.

Professor Rod Griffiths, President of the Faculty of Public Health, believes this is crucial. He told me: 'The most obvious step to take for people who smoke is to stop smoking. If you go on smoking and we get a flu outbreak, you'll be more likely to be worse affected. You may not find a randomized controlled trial that shows this, but what we do know is that smokers get most other respiratory infections so it is just common sense that they will get flu.'

However, the Department of Health is cagey about recommending this, which is strange because they've been running anti-smoking campaigns for some time now. It may be that they don't want bird flu messages to be overly negative, or it may simply be that they are not sure what impact it would have.

'The most obvious step to take for people who smoke is to stop smoking. If you go on smoking and we get a flu outbreak, you'll be more likely to be worse affected.'

A statement for the Department says: 'Smoking in general makes a person more susceptible to respiratory illness as well as having a damaging impact on a person's general health and well-being. That is why we recommend people give up smoking. However, we don't know the impact of smoking on an individual's susceptibility to a pandemic flu virus simply because we don't know what the virus would look like and therefore how it would manifest itself.'

I think it would be good to give up before a pandemic begins. When you do try to quit, your lungs are in a transitional state for a while and some smokers find themselves picking up all kinds of bugs immediately after they stop. If you're going to give up, the message should be to give up now, rather than wait.

If you want to quit, it's a very good idea to tell your GP. He or she can discuss it with you and offer encouragement, and may also prescribe nicotine gum or patches to make the giving-up easier. Many areas have counsellors who will offer support and ideas on how to get over the addiction, either in person or over the telephone. The NHS helpline for anyone who wants to kick the habit is 0800 169 0169. I would give up now. Don't put it off.

ADVICE ON TRAVEL TO SOUTHEAST ASIA

At the time of writing (November 2005), travelling to countries so far affected by bird flu is still a low-risk activity (see Chapter 7). However, if you want to be doubly safe, there are some specific steps you could take. The following measures are recommended by the US Center for Disease Control (CDC) in Atlanta, Georgia:

- *Take with you a first-aid kit containing a thermometer and some alcohol-based hand wipes for regular hand-cleaning.*
- *Research the country's healthcare resources before you go, and find out what you should do in an emergency.*
- *During travel to an affected area, avoid places where live poultry is kept, especially live animal markets and poultry farms.*
- *Don't eat any raw or undercooked poultry products.*
- *Wash your hands carefully and frequently.*
- *If you do become sick, get immediate medical help.*

The CDC also recommends that you monitor your health carefully for ten days after your return. If you fall ill, be sure to tell your doctor that you've been in an area that has had a known avian influenza outbreak. See Chapter 7 for more on this.

PREPARATIONS AT HOME

Flu pandemics in the past have caused a lot of social disruption. In the UK, we already know what this feels like. The fuel crisis of 2002, when tanker drivers went on strike, led to widespread panic buying across the country. Within days, our transport system and food supplies were affected, and the fragility of the infrastructure that we take for granted every day of our lives was exposed.

With this in mind, it's essential that governments, companies, charities and individuals use the time before a pandemic to think about the preparations that need to be made. According to the government's own estimate, around 25 per cent of the workforce would not be at work for at least part of the time that we are in the grip of the pandemic. If it lasts around three months, as experts expect, that means there could be quite a few services affected.

In Britain, there are 3 million key workers, according to the Civil Contingencies Secretariat, which co-ordinates nationwide responses to disasters. The figure of 3 million includes not only doctors, nurses, firemen and police officers, but also those who work in power generation, water supply and telecommunications. We cannot assume that all these services are going to run as smoothly as usual, simply because it is likely that a significant percentage of those 3 million key workers will get flu, and others will stay away from work. Most alarming of all is the fact that Britain already has a shortage of HGV drivers who transport our food around the country, and there is no plan in place to deal with a situation where 10–20 per cent of them would not be available to work.

'It is possible that there will be panic buying in the shops, and this may well occur in the short four-to-eight week phase after the virus goes human and before the pandemic arrives in Britain.'

So what do you need in the home to protect yourself from the worst effects of the disruption? I would suggest that you stock up on some essential supplies now. You don't need crates full of goods – just enough to get you through the first week or so of a pandemic.

It is possible that there will be panic buying in the shops, and this may well occur in the short four-to-eight week phase after the virus goes human and before the pandemic arrives in Britain. Nobody wants to be a panic buyer, but equally no one wants to be caught short without food to give their family. Given the very long shelf life that many food products have these days, it is quite an easy operation to stock up on a few basic provisions.

- Cans of food and non-perishables are particularly useful to store. Eating well is important for your general health, so buy healthy food that is low in fat, salt and sugar but high in fibre.

Cans of baked beans, rice pudding, tinned vegetables or tinned fruit are good. You could also stock dried rice, pasta or pulses. Make sure it is all properly sealed up and you could store it in a box in the garage, or in a garden shed. It might also be worth ensuring you have a well-stocked freezer.

- Have a bottle of water to hand. Some of the big 2-litre bottles of water might be useful, and when they have reached their sell-by date you can replenish them with normal tap water. Our water supplies should continue as normal in the middle of an emergency, but we can't know this for sure.

- One thing we so often overlook is batteries, but how will torches or radios work if there are power cuts? You can also buy battery-operated devices to keep your mobile charged. A stash of candles and some boxes of matches may also be a good bet.

- A medicine kit is essential. If the pharmacies have to close because they are being swamped by people demanding help, it would be good to have your own supplies of medical aids. It is always useful to have aspirin or Nurofen (ibuprofen) in the cupboard, as they can alleviate all kinds of symptoms. Remember that aspirin should not be given to children under the age of sixteen – buy Calpol or child-friendly Nurofen for any younger family members. Some basic pain-relief and a cough linctus will be useful to deal with the symptoms, and a thermometer is essential for checking temperatures.

I went to a supermarket myself to decide what I would put in my emergency store. Everyone would have their own favourites to add, but I thought that the provisions below would easily see me and my family through the first few days of any crisis. In the absence of fresh fruit, veg or meat, you can always fall back on tinned vegetables, dried fruit and tinned meat. This is what I included for my family of four:

12 loo rolls • disinfectant spray for kitchen surfaces • disinfectant liquid for the floor and toilets • a torch plus batteries • dishcloths • 2 boxes of tissues • box of washing powder • light bulbs

and matches • six candles • pack of six soaps • box of teabags • container of dried milk • jar of coffee • large bag of rice • large bag of pasta • bag of sugar • bag of porridge oats • 5-litre bottle of water • 1-litre bottle of orange squash • tin of grapefruit segments • 4 tins of baked beans • tin of corned beef • tin of pork meatballs • 3 tins of different beans (haricots, lentils, black-eyed) • tinned sweetcorn and tinned spinach

The bill came to £37.75. Obviously you could buy far more tins, or far more water, but this shopping filled about three bags and takes up very little room in the corner of our garden shed.

Here are just a few further suggestions to keep you all in optimum health:

- Put a bottle of vitamin C supplements in your food store. These may be useful because no one can guarantee that fresh fruit and veg will be easy to come by if food supplies are disrupted.

- You can store some apples in the shed over winter by wrapping each one individually and putting them in a box. It's what generations did for centuries before we got used to the idea of supermarkets having strawberries all year round.

- Take Dr Carey's advice (see page 154) and store Omega-3 supplements for your family. Cod-liver oil is the alternative, but that's pretty unpalatable for most children.

- I recommend getting hold of some flu masks, but other experts don't necessarily agree with me on this. Read pages 164–166 and make up your own mind.

Keep a list of the essential numbers you may need in a crisis somewhere handy and close to the phone. I would include: NHS Direct (0845 4647), the local council, the local police station, your GP practice, the nearest hospital trust, your local vet (if you have a pet), the local pharmacy, your regional transport office, and, if you have children, the number(s) for their school(s).

Revise your list as we move closer to a pandemic situation,

because some of the emergency helpline numbers won't yet be established. Once there is a pandemic, a special number is likely to be issued for people who are worried that they may have the symptoms. The local council will probably be responsible for the emergency response in your area.

CLAIMS AND QUACKERY

Already I've read news reports about some so-called 'miracle' foods and nutritional products that are said to help you fight off bird flu. Sauerkraut (a German chopped cabbage dish), ginseng, *kimchi* (a south Korean dish of fermented cabbage), zinc tablets, elderberry tea, garlic, broccoli and Brazil nuts are just a few of the items for which anti-viral claims are made.

'Researchers fed kimchi to thirteen chickens that were infected with H5N1 and a week later, eleven of them showed signs of recovery.'

Let's look at *kimchi* and the fantastic hype it has achieved. In November 2005, a report emerged from Seoul National University claiming that this fermented, chopped cabbage contains a bacteria which could combat the disease in chickens. Researchers fed *kimchi* to thirteen chickens that were infected with H5N1 and a week later, eleven of them showed signs of recovery. It was claimed that German sauerkraut could have the same effects and the news led to an immediate rush to buy sauerkraut, with the Sainsbury supermarket chain buying in extra jars of a food which, until then, had a very small market in the UK.

Unfortunately, it is unlikely these cabbage dishes will help human beings. It is impossible to see how lactobacillus, the lactic acid bacteria that seems to have the anti-viral effect in chickens, could help people with a pandemic strain because the disease affects the respiratory tract in humans, rather than the gut as it does in birds. But this story shows how desperate people are to try anything when they see a threat looming on the horizon.

Certainly broccoli, garlic and Brazil nuts are nutritious foods containing essential vitamins and minerals that may help keep you

Disease control research

Dr John Watson, who runs the respiratory diseases department of the Health Protection Agency, is in charge of advising the government about measures that might work during a pandemic. His team has been working extremely hard throughout 2004 and 2005 to assess the different strategies, while studying what is happening with the virus in Southeast Asia.

Talking to me from his office at the HPA headquarters in north London, he explained: 'Exposure is the over-riding factor that matters. Common sense would tell you that the healthier you are, the better the position you'll be in to ward off the infection, although we just don't know how much that is true.' Unfortunately, there is a real shortage of research to show why some people might be very badly affected by a virulent strain, while others escape it completely. There may be genetic factors at play, but currently we just don't know how they may work.

'Even if you take a room full of healthy people, each one will have a different immune system, because of the infections to which they have been exposed in the past,' he explained. 'In relation to flu, we know that your chance of going down with it is almost certainly related to your previous exposures to that, or similar strains of flu. But with a pandemic, the problem is that it's a strain that no one has had exposure to.'

I asked Dr Watson how much public health measures, such as wearing of flu masks, quarantining infected individuals or better personal hygiene, actually reduced the spread of the disease. He said: 'The truth is that we don't have a very good understanding of the extent to which certain actions will ultimately lead to a lower burden of disease in a population as a whole.' If you have a combination of factors such as warm, dry air in summer, with people spending time

(continued over)

outside and also washing their hands properly, perhaps this might be enough to delay the influenza for a while.

   'But really, one needs to fall back on first principles. Given that some people will inevitably fall ill, you would not want them to pass that infection on to someone else.'

---

healthy, but they do not offer miraculous protection against viruses. Similarly, I have been asked about the efficacy of homeopathic and herbal remedies to boost the immune system and fight off infection. You should be aware that there is a great dearth of evidence to show that such therapies work against normal flu. One of the problems facing alternative therapists is that very few studies have been carried out to show whether or not their products or their techniques work. No one can possibly judge if herbal remedies, for example, would help you in a pandemic situation. And if you are already taking other medications, you should talk to your doctor before switching over to any different therapies.

COUGHING AND SNEEZING

The single greatest factor governing whether you catch a dangerous strain of flu will not be your own state of health – it will be the extent of your exposure to the virus. This means that the top priority has to be cutting down on your chances of being in contact with other peoples' germs, and avoiding transmitting them if you are infected yourself.

   How many times have you sat on a train or a bus and got really annoyed when someone sneezed without bothering to use a tissue, or even their hand, to cover their nose? If a pandemic begins, one of the most important public health messages will be about the importance of using a tissue whenever you cough or sneeze. Just one sneeze can send 100,000 viral particles flying through the air. Imagine how important this is going to be in a flu outbreak. You have a virulent virus, capable of being ejected from your nose at more than 80 miles an hour whenever you sneeze. Even if someone is on the other side of the room, that droplet could land on their skin, or their mouth, or even in their eye.

A tissue traps germs, but it must be disposed of properly, because otherwise the virus will live on the tissue and potentially infect others. It's a good idea to keep a small bin (which should be disinfected regularly) in the kitchen for throwing away infected tissues. Cotton handkerchiefs may be more stylish but they are not as hygienic as tissues, and for this reason they are not recommended by most healthcare experts.

The other warning is that anyone who is suffering the symptoms of flu should not be allowed to prepare food. If your work involves food preparation, you should stay at home at the first signs of flu so others can't be infected. If you normally make the meals for the family, pass the responsibility on to someone else if you become ill.

'Just one sneeze can send 100,000 viral particles flying through the air. Imagine how important this is going to be in a flu outbreak.'

This is a big public health issue, even in a normal wintertime. In December 2004, the Health Protection Agency (HPA) was forced to issue an urgent plea for any food handlers who were suffering from colds to stay away from work. They did so because agency staff in northwest England had noticed caterers who were clearly suffering from infections handling food and serving customers in a number of settings, including a sandwich bar, a coffee house and a supermarket café. In one wine bar, they saw a waitress sneeze on her hands without using a handkerchief, then give them a cursory run under a tap, wipe them on a towel and continue to prepare and serve food.

If someone sneezes near you, turn away from them and close your eyes at the same time. Don't rub your eyes, because viral particles can enter through the corner of the eyes and travel down the tear ducts into the body. Try to wash your hands and face as soon as possible (see the handwashing advice on page 167). And, if you're feeling brave, ask the 'sneezer' to use a tissue next time.

SHOULD YOU WEAR A FLU MASK?

If one image has stuck in our minds from the SARS epidemic of 2003, it is of a nation going to work wearing flu masks. It seems the whole of Singapore suddenly took to wearing them when they heard about the threat. Some fashion designers even tried to turn the craze to their advantage by producing attractively coloured ones.

Although you may think that wearing a mask is an obvious way to reduce your risk of getting flu, there is very little evidence to suggest it works. Health experts in Britain actually think the opposite may be true – that wearing a mask gives people a false sense of security and may mean that they are less likely to follow other procedures that would limit their exposure to the virus.

Dr Jonathan van Tam, a consultant epidemiologist with the HPA, told me: 'This is an emotive issue. People feel that it will protect them against anything that is airborne. We've been investigating the role of masks for the government, and there are actually pitfalls to wearing them. The biggest danger is that they could be worn for long periods of time, and the germs will be carried around with them.' The virus can live for up to eight hours on soft materials, and anyone taking the mask off when they get home risks getting it on their fingers.

He said that most healthcare staff who wear surgical masks for infection control have special training to make sure they are fitted properly. The most protective masks of all, also known as respirators, can restrict breathing so you have to take breaks in between using them. In Britain, masks are classified according to their FFP factor. The most effective are the FFP3 or FFP2 types, which filter out 99 per cent or 95 per cent of particles respectively (overseas, these are known as N99 or N95 masks). There are also much more simple surgical masks, which are made of paper and can be tied on behind the ears; these are the kind that were worn by members of the public during the SARS outbreak but they don't have any FFP factor and it is unclear how many particles they would keep out during a flu pandemic.

At present the British Department of Health is only recommending the proper FFP3 masks for staff who are dealing very closely with infected patients. The government is not convinced that the mass use of masks would help much, because they suspect many people would not use them properly. However, other countries seem to be considering relying heavily on masks. France has bought more than 200 million masks as part of its flu pandemic plan. The Hong Kong government is giving its citizens clear advice on how to safely put on and take off a mask, without risk of infection. On their Department of Health website (see page 218), there is advice on how to change masks without touching the part that may be infected with the virus.

The Center for Disease Control (CDC) in America has also addressed the issue. Like the HPA, the CDC does not believe that masks are going to limit transmission of disease across a whole community, but they don't completely disregard them. Their guidance states if someone is symptomatic and cannot stay at home during their illness, consideration should be given to having them wear a mask in public places when they may have close contact with other people.

'The government is not convinced that the mass use of masks would help much, because they suspect many people would not use them properly.'

Personally, I would want some kind of protection if I had to travel by public transport during a pandemic, and that protection would be an FFP2 mask, or respirator, which has a valve in the middle so you can exhale quite easily. But it is wise to remember Dr van Tam's advice and make sure you dispose of the mask safely. At the moment, the best way of getting hold of flu masks is buying them over the Internet.

I would also want to wear one if I had to attend any kind of large gathering where I was close to others, but I wouldn't want to wear one at home for long. I doubt they would protect the rest of the family, because if you became infectious, the viral particles would be widespread around the house, particularly on surfaces, and you would still exhale some of the germs through the valve.

If you have young children or a baby, it certainly is worth getting some masks in store, so that you can avoid breathing germs over them while feeding them. The CDC recommends that masks should be given to nursing mothers if they develop flu-like symptoms, in order to avoid breathing the germs onto the baby.

KEEPING IT CLEAN

If you want to cut down on your risk of picking up the virus, it's important to understand where germs lurk in the home or in a workplace.

Research by the Health Protection Agency suggests that on stainless steel, a flu virus can survive for between 24 and 48 hours. You will be able to pick it up from hard surfaces like desks, computer keyboards and phones long after the infected person has gone. On softer surfaces, such as a sofa, clothes or a newspaper or book, it is closer to eight hours. The one piece of good news is that the virus appears to last for only a few minutes on your skin, so regular washing can be an invaluable self-help measure.

'You will be able to pick it up from hard surfaces like desks, computer keyboards and phones long after the infected person has gone.'

Viruses are sensitive to both heat and humidity. The flu virus in a piece of infected meat would be destroyed by normal cooking. It is also harder for the virus to survive in dry rather than humid air. It's generally more humid indoors than out, which is why winter is such a bad time for flu, because everyone is bundled up together inside.

Keeping surfaces clean and hygienic will be essential in a pandemic. You don't need to buy sophisticated, super-strength products or special anti-bacterial cleaning agents. Normal disinfectant, such as Dettol, will kill any virus contained in droplets on surfaces very quickly.

Remember to clean the following carefully:

• Door handles (these are often overlooked)

- All kitchen surfaces
- Bathroom surfaces, particularly toilet seats (many people touch them as they get on and off)
- Toys that your children are handling a lot
- Computer keyboards
- The phone, especially the mouthpiece

Once you have cleaned surfaces, remember to wash the cloths properly. A normal machine cycle will be perfectly adequate for destroying any germs. While you are cleaning you can wear rubber gloves if you wish, but these will have to be washed too. It may be better simply to wash your hands well for 30 seconds (see below) with soap and water – and remember not to touch your face until you have washed your hands.

'We touch our mouth, nose, eyes or ears – the entry points for disease – between one and three times every five minutes and most of the time we're not even conscious of doing so.'

WASH YOUR HANDS

Handwashing is a procedure that nearly everyone is taught as a child, but it's amazing how many people forget about it, or choose to take shortcuts, once they grow up. It's estimated that up to one fifth of all adults don't wash their hands after going to the toilet and fewer than half of us wash our hands after we've sneezed into them, so be careful who you shake hands with, even at the best of times.

In a pandemic, handwashing is going to become imperative – in some cases, the difference between life and death. It's difficult to emphasize enough just how much thorough handwashing will matter. We touch our mouth, nose, eyes or ears – the entry points for disease – between one and three times every five minutes and most of the time we're not even conscious of doing so. More than three quarters of all diseases are spread via hands and in a flu pandemic, hand-to-mouth or hand-to-nose transmission is just as big a risk as airborne viral particles from someone coughing directly onto you.

You should wash your hands every time you cough or sneeze, even if you've used a tissue. If someone at home or at work is sick, this habit will become even more critical. If you have children, teach them now about the importance of handwashing. Tell them to spend 30 seconds rubbing their soapy hands, and try to make it fun, as if it's a game. Here are the seven steps to clean hands:

- Wet your hands under clean, warm, running water.

- Apply liquid soap or use a bar of soap. There's no need to resort to expensive anti-bacterial products. Make sure any suds or water can drain off the soap when you put it down.

- Make a lather and rub all over your hands and exposed parts of your wrists and lower arms.

- Every part of the hand should be rubbed. Interlace your fingers so that the bits in between are cleaned, and make sure the knuckles get covered.

- Keep rubbing your hands for 30 seconds.

- Rinse under cold running water.

- Dry your hands with a paper towel or an air dryer. At home, ensure that towels are dry, as damp towels encourage bacteria to breed.

If you don't have access to soap and water, alcohol-based wipes are a good method of cleaning hands. In a pandemic, you may want to carry some wipes with you so that you can clean your hands regularly when you are out and about.

PROTECTING BABIES AND YOUNG CHILDREN

When it comes to caring for the very young, pandemic flu presents healthcare staff with all kinds of challenges. Infants are vulnerable to flu, and can be prone to serious complications such as pneumonia or dehydration, when they become too sick to drink enough fluids. There is also an increased risk of bronchiolitis, an infection of the lungs.

Unfortunately, the anti-viral medications Tamiflu and Relenza cannot be given to children under the age of one, because it is not known whether they could harm the developing brain; for this reason, they are also not recommended for breastfeeding mothers. If a breastfeeding mother contracted pandemic flu, her best course would be to switch the baby onto formula milk so that she could take Tamiflu or whatever medication the doctor recommended. She should also wear a flu mask in the vicinity of her baby to try and avoid passing on the infection – but chances are she would be feeling so ill that a partner or relative would have to take over the bottle-feeding and baby care for the duration of the illness.

Infection control has to be top priority for anyone with a child under the age of one. Parents and those caring for babies should follow these five basic rules religiously:

- Cover your nose and mouth completely when coughing or sneezing.

- Use a tissue to contain the germs then dispose of it in the nearest bin after use.

- Wash your hands regularly with soap or an alcohol-based wipe, especially after contact with respiratory secretions or any material that may be contaminated.

- Try to avoid touching your eyes, nose or mouth, since germs can spread in this way.

- Keep your baby and yourself away from people who are coughing and sneezing as much as you possibly can.

If your baby or young child does develop symptoms – a fever of 100°F (37°C) or higher, respiratory symptoms, or if they appear less responsive than normal – call your doctor or NHS Direct straight away.

It's a good idea to buy a digital thermometer, because they are easier to use on a small child. Make sure you have lots of pain relief, such as Calpol, in your medicine cupboard and make your child drink as much liquid as possible.

ADVICE FOR ASTHMATICS

Anyone with asthma, young or old, is eligible for the normal, seasonal flu vaccine administered by GPs, and it is highly recommended that they get this. It's understandable that parents of asthmatic children in particular will be worried about their welfare in the event of a bird flu pandemic. I asked Dr Peter Openshaw, the consultant in respiratory medicine who wrote the foreword to this book, for his advice.

'It's true that patients with asthma tend to be more susceptible to viral colds, and suffer exacerbations as a result,' he said. 'The standard advice is that if you have asthma and a cold or flu, you should double the inhaler dose for the period of illness. The inhalers are very safe so increasing treatment is a good idea (especially if only for a week or two).'

It may also be sensible to keep a few spare Ventolin inhalers in your medicine cupboard as these are likely to be in short supply if pharmacists are busy during a pandemic.

SCHOOL MAY BE OUT

Should you take your children out of school once you know Britain is in the middle of a pandemic? This is a very difficult decision because children can be highly contagious, and a viral infection can whip round a school in no time at all. Every winter we see contagious stomach bugs or respiratory infections doing the rounds. At present, the government has said it will leave it to local education authorities to make the decision about closing schools in the event of a pandemic, but this doesn't help you much in trying to assess the situation.

I suspect that many parents will automatically withdraw their children from school once a pandemic starts. Head teachers will have to decide whether or not to keep the school open if both pupils and teachers start to fall sick. For this reason, it might be sensible to plan ahead once we are in Phase 5 of a pandemic alert – when it has spread broadly across several countries but not reached Britain (see page 150). What would you do if your child was off school for weeks on end? Could you share the childcare with your partner? Would your employer let you work from home or take time off? Could you share childcare with a friend in an emergency?

One difficulty may be that during a pandemic, family members infect each other, so within the space of a few days, both parents and children could go down with the flu. Everyone knows how common it is for a particularly nasty cold bug to spread its way across the family – and pandemic flu would be no different. There is nothing you can do to prevent this happening, other than trying to maintain rigorous handwashing and hygiene procedures to cut down on the risk of you all taking to your beds at once.

If schools close down, do you have the resources to do a bit of home education? There are many Internet sites which offer opportunities for learning, so that you could embark on a history or geography project with your child. It's even conceivable that if there was a mass closure of schools, the government might broadcast educational programmes during the day, although there are no plans to do this at the moment.

'Once they have been infected, both children and adults will carry the antibodies against the virus, should it return in a second wave of the pandemic.'

I think it's also important to remember that if your child is infected, it is overwhelmingly likely that they will be laid low by the bug for up to a week and then make a full recovery. At that point, it would be sensible for them to go back to school. Once they have been infected, both children and adults will carry the antibodies against the virus, should it return in a second wave of the pandemic.

PREPARATIONS AT WORK

Have you asked your employer about their plans for a flu pandemic? If you work for a large organization that is listed as an 'essential service', such as British Telecom, they will already be producing a preparedness plan. Someone within the company will be co-ordinating the different responses so that once an alert is declared by the World Health Organization, the plan will go into action.

But it is becoming clear that many companies are completely unprepared for a pandemic because they see it as a distant event. Bruce Mann, the head of the Civil Contingencies Secretariat, the part of Whitehall responsible for emergency planning, warned at a conference organized by the Union Bank of Switzerland in November 2005 that businesses needed to become more engaged in planning.

'The primary focus for us, in everything we do, is about saving lives,' he said. 'But of course there will be issues about keeping the essential services running. If people are off work – if important people can no longer come to work – what do we do? Once influenza comes here it will take only two to three weeks to spread across the country.'

He said that a particular problem was that 'plans tend to be written around middle and junior management'. They did not concentrate enough either on the senior directors at the very top of the company or, he added, on the essential workers who keep services going but are lower down the pecking order. Mr Mann, who is the UK's most senior emergency planning official, said that there was often one person within a company who might be technically very important, for example keeping the building running, but who would be overlooked by the plans.

The Health and Safety Executive is expected to issue new guidance to businesses in December 2005 which will tell both employees and employers how to equip themselves for a pandemic. But meanwhile, here are some questions to put to your employers:

- Have you got a plan for dealing with a flu pandemic?

- Has the company or organization looked carefully at the issue of staffing? Perhaps they would consider the use of temporary staff to overcome severe shortages.

- If a pandemic comes, will it be possible for you to work from home for some of that time? Would they consider making it easier for employees to do home-working via the Internet?

- Would the company be prepared to stagger working hours, so that employees would not have to travel on public transport during the rush hour?

- Has the organization bought any anti-viral medication or flu masks and, if so, who is going to get them?

MOVING TO AN ISOLATED SPOT

It is impossible to count the number of times in recent months I have been told by friends that they will leave London as soon there is a pandemic alert and live in the countryside for a few months, until the worst blows over. Are we likely to see a great exodus out of our towns and cities once the warning is given that we are just days or weeks away from a pandemic? And if you are tempted to leave, would it actually do any good?

'Are we likely to see a great exodus out of our towns and cities once the warning is given that we are just days or weeks away from a pandemic?'

Angela McLean is an eminent epidemiologist at Oxford University, where she heads its Institute for Emergent Infections for Humans. She caused controversy within the medical community when she admitted on a BBC 'Panorama' programme in October 2005 that she planned to leave the city with her children if there was an outbreak.

I asked Professor McLean why she thought it would help to take her children out of school and move to an isolated spot in the countryside for three months. She replied: 'So my children would be removed from social contact with other children but they could still get out and do stuff.' And she added: 'You cannot completely remove yourself socially, unless you own a private island with its own veg garden, but you can greatly reduce the amount of social contact you have and correspondingly the likelihood you will be infected.' But Professor McLean explained that she would only take this action if there was a strain of pandemic flu that had very serious consequences in children, and she pointed out that most influenza is mild in children.

Many people may be similarly tempted to leave their urban areas. After all, if the greatest risk factor is exposure to the disease, moving to an isolated region should cut back exposure and might therefore cut back risk. But in a pandemic situation, there won't actually be any part of the country that is free of the disease. Disease-mapping work carried out by the Health Protection Agency suggests there will not be a single village without cases of pandemic flu.

Imagine moving to a country village for the duration of a pandemic. What would happen? For a start, you might not know many people to call on for help. You would not be near a major hospital if any of the family developed complications. If there was a food or petrol shortage, you would be further away from supplies. Mostly importantly, the flu would still reach your village at some point, even if you felt a long way away from civilization. Would it really be any better?

I think that before there is a mass exodus to the country during a pandemic alert, it would be sensible for people to find out more about the nature of the disease. Once it starts to spread easily between people, doctors will be able to judge if it is particularly dangerous for children. In 1957, for example, the flu pandemic was extremely contagious among children, but very few died – most of the mortality was seen in older adults.

THE TROUBLE WITH QUARANTINE

It is possible that people who have been exposed to pandemic flu may be asked to stay at home to prevent them from spreading it – and if they refuse to comply, the police could be asked to enforce quarantine. But this is a step which the government is loathe to take. Compulsory quarantine would only work in the initial four to six weeks of the pandemic, because after that the disease would be widespread, and it would be impossible for the police to impose it on so many.

If you are asked to stay at home because you have been exposed to someone with the virus, the main challenge for you is going to be keeping mentally strong enough to cope with days and possibly weeks inside. It sounds so easy, even appealing, to talk of spending time at home – but it's a different issue when you don't have any choice. We know that quarantine can have serious psychological consequences. In March 2003, when Canada was struck by SARS, more than 15,000 people were placed in quarantine. A follow-up study of 129 of them carried out at the University of Toronto showed a high prevalence of psychological distress. More than one quarter of them suffered the equivalent of post-traumatic stress disorder, and the longer the quarantine lasted, the worse the effect.

Be aware that quarantine can be very stressful, and that you would need to remain mentally resilient for this. Think about the impact of barricading yourself at home for weeks on end, with or without children. Would you have the resourcefulness to cope? Could you take up a hobby to occupy yourself through some very difficult days? Could you find activities to entertain the rest of the family?

> **'Think about the impact of barricading yourself at home for weeks on end, with or without children. Would you have the resourcefulness to cope?'**

If this sounds alarmist, it isn't intended to be. It is simply an observation that, based on the Canadian experience, quarantine can be a very distressing time and you might need support from others to get through it.

YOUR MENTAL HEALTH

Panic and anxiety are bound to be widespread when the world first hears that a virulent strain of bird flu has acquired the ability to become a human form. There is likely to be a great deal of alarm, even hysteria, among those who are worried they won't be able to get medical help or even food supplies.

For this reason, it's very important to stay as calm and collected as possible. Remember that the vast majority of people who are infected will suffer nothing more than a very nasty bout of flu.

Your mental state will matter because it can have an impact on your hormones and therefore on your physical health, but it also matters because it affects those around you. Panic is as infectious as flu. If you have children, it's essential that you stay calm for them because they need to see that adults can cope with this.

Yoga and meditation can be excellent ways of relieving stress levels. Others find that simply going for a walk, or listening to some music can help. Everyone has their own way of coping with anxiety, and you should find time to do something that will be therapeutic. It might be something constructive, such as taking up a new hobby or doing something practical like DIY or cooking.

When people panic, strange things happen. They can suffer a racing pulse, a dry mouth, feelings of aggression, jaw pain and even hallucinations. Being physically active will help keep some of these symptoms at bay, however worried you feel.

'Panic is as infectious as flu. If you have children, it's essential that you stay calm for them because they need to see that adults can cope with this.'

You would think that in wartime, it must have been very common for people to experience anxiety, depression and generally poor mental health. In fact, the opposite was true during World War II. The mental health of the nation actually appeared to improve, possibly because when a society faces a common enemy, concerns about oneself seem less important, and the mind focuses instead on the immediate threat.

Paul Salkovskis, professor of clinical psychology at the Institute of Psychiatry in London and an expert in anxiety disorders, said that there is very little evidence from previous flu pandemics to show how it affected people's mental health. 'We know that when society faces an external threat such as a terrorist attack you can often see a drop in the levels of anxiety disorders and depression, as more general worries fade into the background,' he explained. 'But it might be different with an infectious agent, and we have seen people in Britain worried over food scares. There can also be a high level of distrust over government messages, as we saw in the reaction to the issue of MMR [the scare about the measles, mumps and rubella vaccine].'

THE DIFFICULTIES FACING HEALTHCARE WORKERS

If you are a nurse or doctor confronted by a patient who is desperately worried about the prospect of pandemic flu, what can you say to them? At the moment, there is no detailed guidance for healthcare staff about how to explain to people the information they may need.

The Department of Health is preparing guidance for staff but, at present, the best you could do is refer to the government's own patient leaflets, which explain why people are worried about a pandemic and how they are planning for one. The British Medical Association is advising doctors to stress to patients that currently, the H5N1 strain exists in birds but that it has not become a fully humanized strain.

However, if you care for patients with chronic conditions, such as heart disease, diabetes or compromised immunity, the more detailed information you need will simply not be forthcoming for a while. It is expected that during 2006, the government will roll out an information campaign spelling out some of the public health messages that are included here. In the meantime, it is a good idea for those with chronic conditions to talk to their specialists and the organizations dedicated to their condition, such as the British Heart Foundation, for a clearer idea of the help they might need during a flu pandemic.

'When the strain of flu becomes a human pandemic form, it is likely that scientists will see a particular pattern of symptoms emerging, such as severe coughing and a high temperature.'

WHAT TO DO IF YOU GO DOWN WITH PANDEMIC FLU

The symptoms of influenza can be very wide-ranging, and it can sometimes just seem like a bad cold. The first signs might be a fever, a cough, sore throat, bad headache, a streaming nose, aching muscles, a sore neck or very tired eyes. When the strain of flu becomes a human pandemic form, it is likely that scientists will see a particular pattern of symptoms emerging, such as severe coughing and a high temperature.

If you become unwell, it will be important for you to recognize symptoms at an early stage, but not to exaggerate them. This is what I would suggest:

- If you have the symptoms of flu, take your temperature and write it down.
- Ring your GP practice or NHS Direct for advice, giving as accurate a description as possible of the symptoms.
- If they ask you to come and collect medication, see if a friend can go for you, if that is allowed; if not, go yourself.
- Go to bed with plenty of fluids and hot water with lemon and honey, plus some painkillers.
- Get a friend or partner to tell your employers that you won't be coming in.
- At all costs, avoid coughing or sneezing over those around you.
- Wash your hands frequently to avoid passing germs on to others. Keep hand wipes by the bed.
- Stay in one room as much as possible.
- Write down your symptoms as they develop.
- Take the medication as directed by your GP.

AND HERE IS WHAT YOU SHOULD NOT DO:

- Don't carry on going to work; your flu will get worse and you'll infect others.
- Don't cough or sneeze without using a tissue.
- Don't go out shopping or meet friends if you have any flu-like symptoms.
- Don't take any form of exercise – it will make your temperature higher and drain the energy you need to fight the virus.
- Don't demand a home visit from your GP when they will be inundated by calls.
- Don't sit close to others while you have symptoms – keep your distance.

- Don't try to save some of your medication for others because it might not work properly on you if you don't take the full course.

- Don't touch door handles or hard surfaces in the kitchen without asking someone to disinfect them afterwards.

- Don't smoke. You will exacerbate the symptoms.

- Don't drink alcohol. It will make recovery much harder.

When one of your family or a friend goes down with flu, there is a limited amount you can do for them. If you have already had the flu yourself, it will be much easier because you won't be worried about catching it. If you haven't had it, you will have to try and limit your exposure to them. You will have to bring them food and drink while they are in bed, but ask them to turn away so they can't breathe the germs over you. Make sure, as ever, that you thoroughly wash your hands after any contact. Viruses can be carried on clothes so if the patient touched your clothes, make sure you change and wash them as normal.

'When caring for flu patients, bring them lots of hot and cold drinks, offer painkillers and keep checking that their condition isn't deteriorating.'

When caring for flu patients, bring them lots of hot and cold drinks, offer painkillers and keep checking that their condition isn't deteriorating. The main problem you should watch out for is signs of difficulty in breathing. This isn't simply about having a bad cough – it's about the breathing become very laboured to the point where the patient starts to feel they can't get enough air into the lungs. You may also see a blue tinge around the lips. At this point, ring your GP practice or NHS Direct for help.

If someone has a heart condition, watch out for signs that they are getting pains in the chest, arms or legs, which could indicate a heart attack. Another warning sign is if the patient starts to cough up blood or large amounts of yellow or green phlegm. In both cases, get urgent medical help.

These are the main messages for anyone with flu:

• Go to bed and get as much rest as possible.

• Keep warm, but don't get overheated.

• Make sure you drink plenty of fluids.

• Take painkillers such as paracetamol to relieve headaches and fever.

You can go back to work as soon as you feel well again. Be aware that you may feel very tired for a couple of weeks afterwards, but this can happen after normal flu as well. Just eat healthily, try not to get run down or stressed and get as much sleep as you possibly can.

IN CONCLUSION

These days, we are used to receiving one-to-one treatment when we fall ill. We are consumers of healthcare, rather than passive recipients of it. How then will we cope when faced with an infection for which there may be no one-to-one care available because the virus will have affected 25 per cent or more of the population? Can we show the forbearance that was seen in the 1918 pandemic when people suffered such hardship in the middle of a war, with no access to medication or intensive care?

It is understandable that people will want to protect themselves and their families from the H5N1 virus. But what do you do for those who live alone, or those who are elderly or frail? I would like to see the government set up a system whereby those who had no one close to care for them could call on emergency help near by. Everyone has neighbours, and we need to think about how people are going to help each other in a pandemic flu situation.

This chapter has tried to explain that, however frightening pandemic flu may be, there are steps you can take to prepare for it. But the best protection of all will always be the measures that strengthen the whole of society – and in the case of flu, they consist of a series of very simple steps, such as handwashing to stop the spread of germs. It remains to be seen whether the public can be convinced that they are a good idea.

Never before have we had so much early warning about the spread of an influenza virus – and never before have we had so much opportunity to prepare for it, using all our resources and our common sense.

A BRIEF HISTORY OF BIRD FLU

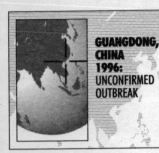
GUANGDONG, CHINA 1996: UNCONFIRMED OUTBREAK

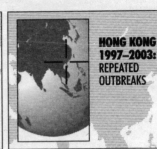
HONG KONG 1997–2003: REPEATED OUTBREAKS

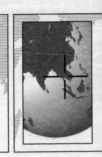

H5N1 proliferation

1996
• An outbreak of disease in geese in the Guangdong province of southern China may have been the first cases of the lethal subtype H5N1. Not confirmed.

MAY 1997
• Hong Kong doctors see the first patient, a young boy, die of H5N1 in May.

DECEMBER 1997
• Eighteen people in Hong Kong are found to have the infection after being in poultry markets. All receive medical attention but six of them die. The authorities stamp out the disease by culling 1.5 million chickens within a 48-hour period.

2001, 2002
• Hong Kong suffers two smaller outbreaks of H5N1, and again has to cull poultry.

FEBRUARY 2003
• H5N1 reappears in Hong Kong after a family visits China. One member of the family survives, but two others die. One family member dies in China.

The first human case of H5N1 bird flu was reported in 1997, but by July 2004 the virus was endemic in poultry in Asia and had killed more than 30 people.

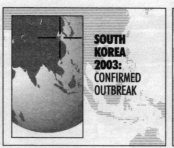
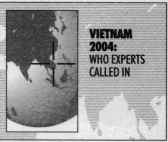

THAILAND NOVEMBER 2003: UNCONFIRMED OUTBREAK

SOUTH KOREA 2003: CONFIRMED OUTBREAK

VIETNAM 2004: WHO EXPERTS CALLED IN

NOVEMBER 2003

• Chickens start to die on farms in Thailand. Authorities deny it is H5N1.

DECEMBER 2003

• Outbreak among chickens on a farm south of Seoul, South Korea.

JANUARY 2004

• Vietnam calls in the World Health Organization (WHO) experts for help following the deaths of eight people. Japan reports avian flu among its poultry. Thailand reports its first human case of bird flu.

FEBRUARY 2004

• Indonesia admits that it has had outbreaks dating back to the previous August.
• Cambodia, China and Laos bring in culling measures after discovering infected poultry stocks, while UN warns that culling is not enough to eradicate the disease.

JULY 2004

• Influenza expert Dr Robert Webster and colleagues warn that bird flu is now endemic in poultry in Asia, and many ducks are asymptomatic carriers of the disease.

By the end of 2004, the virus had begun to spread westward and the World Health Organization warned that a pandemic could occur.

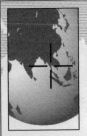 **KELANTAN REGION, MALAYSIA 2004:** UNCONFIRMED CASES IN BIRDS

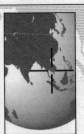 **CAMBODIA FEBRUARY 2005:** FIRST CASE REPORTED

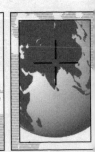

H5N1 proliferation

• The virus infects more people in Vietnam. Long delays in getting the specimens analysed in laboratories abroad.

• New outbreaks in poultry discovered in Ayutthaya and Pathumthani in Thailand and in Anhui, China.

AUGUST 2004

• Cases in birds found in two fighting cocks in Kampung Pasir, in Kelantan region of Malaysia.

• Two young sisters and a third person die in southern Vietnam.

SEPTEMBER 2004

• Several deaths in Thailand, including a thirteen-year-old boy and an eleven-year-old girl.

• WHO warns that bird flu is now a crisis of global importance. First probable human-to-human transmission in Thailand, as mother dies after contracting H5N1 from her daughter.

OCTOBER 2004

• Thailand brings in a tough surveillance and culling policy to try to eradicate the virus. 80 Bengal tigers die in a Bangkok zoo.

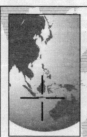

WESTERN CHINA, MAY 2005: OUTBREAK IN MIGRATORY BIRDS

INDONESIA JULY 2005: REGION'S FIRST HUMAN FATALITY

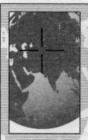

KAZAKHSTAN & MONGOLIA AUGUST 2005: OUTBREAK IN BIRDS CONFIRMED

NOVEMBER 2004

• WHO expert Klaus Stohr tells countries that they need to start preparing for a pandemic.

JANUARY 2005

• Vietnam suffers a terrible explosion of H5N1 cases in birds, affecting 33 out of 64 cities nationwide. More than 1.2m poultry have to be culled.

FEBRUARY 2005

• Cambodia reports its first case of bird flu when a Cambodian woman dies while visiting Vietnam.

MAY 2005

• Migratory birds start to die at Qinghai Lake Nature Reserve in western China. H5N1 is confirmed weeks later after delays caused by red tape.

JULY 2005

• Indonesia suffers its first confirmed human fatality, in Jakarta.
• Philippines reports its first case of flu in poultry.

AUGUST 2005

• Outbreak in bird populations is confirmed in Kazakhstan and Mongolia,

The first case of H5N1 in the EU was found in October 2005, just as the international community was beginning to take action to stop the spread of the disease.

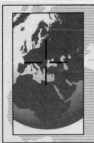

ROMANIA
OCTOBER
2005:
FIRST CASES
IN CHICKENS

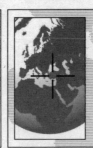

TURKEY
OCTOBER
2005:
LETHAL STRAIN
DETECTED IN
BIRDS

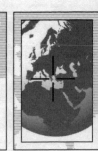

H5N1 proliferation

suggesting that wild birds may be spreading the virus west from Asia.

• A further case in poultry is found in western Russia.

SEPTEMBER 2005

• US President George W. Bush announces a new international partnership to address the threat of avian and pandemic influenza. He also puts more money into vaccine research, as a leaked plan shows US would not be well protected in a pandemic.

OCTOBER 2005

• Romania reports its first cases of bird flu in chickens in the village of Ciamurlia, part of the Danube delta.

• Tests on turkeys on farms in Kiziksa, Turkey, are confirmed to show the lethal strain.

• The Greek island of Inousses becomes the first place in the European Union to have a confirmed case of H5N1.

• China admits it is facing a grave threat from the disease, as thousands of birds succumb to it in Inner Mongolia.

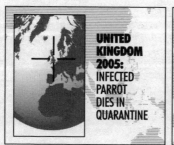

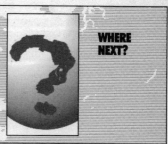

INOUSSES, GREECE OCTOBER 2005: FIRST CONFIRMED CASE IN THE EU

UNITED KINGDOM 2005: INFECTED PARROT DIES IN QUARANTINE

WHERE NEXT?

• A parrot dies in quarantine in the UK after being infected with H5N1 by finches imported from Taiwan.

NOVEMBER 2005

• WHO holds an international meeting so that experts can discuss strategies for controlling the spread of bird flu and limiting the threat of a human pandemic.

• Two-day international emergency planning exercise takes place in Europe to establish just how individual countries would cope in the event of a flu pandemic.

• China confirms its first three human cases of bird flu.

By the end of 2005 the world had woken up to the threat of bird flu, but no one could say with certainty where it would spread to next.

QUESTIONS & ANSWERS

THE VIRUS

What is bird flu?

Bird flu, or avian influenza, is a viral disease that causes illness in many species of birds. It's been around for more than 100 years. There are fifteen different types of bird flu.

Is it the same thing as H5N1?

H5N1 is the particular strain of bird flu which is currently causing worldwide concern. It is a strain that has proved lethal to poultry and has infected some people.

What does H5N1 stand for?

H5N1 is the scientific name for the bird flu virus and denotes the subtype to which the virus belongs. 'H' stands for haemagglutinin, which is a protein that helps the virus attach to a cell. 'N' stands for neuraminidase, which is a protein that allows the virus to leave a host cell and go on to infect other cells. For more information, see page 28.

Why should we be so worried about this particular strain of the flu virus?

H5N1 bird flu has shown an ability to jump from birds into several other species – for example, we know it has infected pigs, cats and humans. This makes it quite unusual. So far there have been 125 human cases, all of whom were infected with the disease after coming into contact with chickens and ducks, and 64 of whom have died. This is worrying, as most animal viruses never affect humans. The problem is that humans have no immunity to animal viruses, so they can hit us hard.

I'm confused – is bird flu the same as SARS?

No. These are two different diseases. Bird flu is caused by a virus that is quite different from the micro-organism, known as a coronavirus, that causes SARS (severe acute respiratory syndrome).

A few years ago everyone was worried about SARS becoming a pandemic, but that didn't happen. Why should we believe the hype about bird flu?

The SARS outbreak could have been extremely nasty, but it transpired that although it was lethal, the coronavirus that caused SARS was very inefficient at leaping from person to person. Bird flu is more dangerous because we know it jumps easily between species, and we know that influenza viruses can be lethal, and can spread fast as people cough and sneeze out the viral particles. There is general scientific agreement that this is the biggest health threat facing the world, and the consensus among doctors and scientists is that the risks are real and must be tackled.

If the authorities have known about the dangers of the H5N1 strain of bird flu since 1997, why has it only become such a big deal in the media in the past year? Why all the fuss now?

Scientists have known about this strain of bird flu since the first infections occurred in Hong Kong in 1997 (see page 37), but it has taken the media a while to wake up to the threat, partly because throughout 2003 and 2004 it was seen as a problem facing Southeast Asia. Now we know that bird flu is a problem affecting the entire globe.

How is bird flu spread?

Many millions of migratory birds and wildfowl carry the disease, and some species of duck are able to carry the virus without showing any symptoms at all. Illegal bird smuggling and the movement of domestic birds has also helped spread the disease across different countries. Birds pass the virus on through their droppings, feathers, saliva and breath. If an infected duck or other water bird uses the same pond or stretch of water as other birds, the infection can be passed on through faeces or shed feathers in the water.

How do humans catch bird flu?

The people who have caught bird flu so far all appear to have had close contact with infected, live birds. Most of the human cases caught the virus when they were preparing chickens for slaughter, but some contracted it by handling infected birds.

Can it pass between people?

The good news is that so far there has not been any scientifically proven human-to-human transmission. All the confirmed human cases so far have been from birds to people. There have been reports of human-to-human transmission in some Asian countries, but these are all unconfirmed.

When will bird flu become a human disease, capable of spreading from one person to another?

This is the million-dollar question. There is simply no way of predicting when the virus will mutate to become an infection that can be easily transmitted between people. However, most experts think this will happen at some point over the next two years.

Why do scientists think this particular virus is likely to develop the ability to spread between humans?

It is in the nature of the flu virus to mutate regularly. This is how some previous flu pandemics have begun. All that is needed is for someone with human flu to also catch H5N1 bird flu from an infected bird and the virus could mutate in such a way that it combines the human flu's ability to spread with H5N1's severe symptoms. Alternatively, the bird flu virus could gradually adapt and jump the species barrier by itself. H5N1 presents a huge risk for humans simply because it is already so widespread in birds.

Are there other examples of diseases that have jumped from animals to humans?

Past flu viruses have made the leap from animal to

human, in particular the Spanish flu that killed tens of millions of people in 1918-19. In addition, it is now accepted that HIV (the virus that leads to AIDS) originally spread from animals to humans. Recent studies have revealed that SARS may have spread from bats, and the UK outbreaks of Creutzfeldt-Jakob Disease (CJD) in the 1990s were directly linked to the incidence of Bovine Spongiform Encephalopathy (BSE – also known as 'Mad Cow Disease') in cattle.

Is it just birds, or do other animals carry this disease?

Several species other than birds have been found to carry the bird flu virus. Pigs in Indonesia have caught H5N1, which is worrying as they can also carry the human flu virus and could act as 'mixing vessels' for the two viruses, allowing them to form a new version of flu which could spread easily between people. Tigers and cats have also been infected, and cats are known to be able to infect other cats.

What makes the bird flu virus mutate?

Scientists know that all flu viruses, even the 'normal' human flu, mutate regularly. In fact, the flu virus mutates every time it replicates. Flu viruses are very unstable and make imperfect copies of themselves, allowing different genetic variations to crop up very quickly.

When the H5N1 virus mutates, will it be deadly?

We don't yet know. Often when a flu virus mutates, there is a trade-off – it may change to become more transmissible within a species but at the same time it may become less virulent. There would be no point in a virus killing all its victims within two days, as it would not be able to spread very far. But if H5N1 does become a human disease with little mutation, it will be bad for us because we have no immunity to any H5 strain of flu.

What is the difference between a pandemic and an epidemic?

A pandemic affects many people over a wide geographical area while an epidemic affects many people in one area or community. A pandemic is effectively an epidemic that has spread over several continents.

SYMPTOMS

Isn't flu just like a very nasty cold?

No. Colds and influenza do have some similar symptoms as they are both respiratory illnesses, but they are not the same and are caused by different viruses. Flu is a much more serious condition. What we call a cold is a relatively minor illness and symptoms are usually confined to the upper respiratory tract (even if you do feel generally unwell when you have a cold). A very bad cold can feel like flu but it will not result in the serious health problems that can result from a flu infection. When someone has flu, their entire body is likely to be affected and they can develop serious health problems.

How does normal human flu kill people?

Normal flu can be lethal for the very young and the very old, those whose immune system is weak or those who have chronic health problems. Sometimes when a person is infected with flu, complications can develop and patients can die of the pneumonia that follows. Seasonal human flu kills around 12,000 people in the UK in an average year.

Why would pandemic flu be worse than seasonal flu?

With a pandemic strain of flu (which is what scientists worry H5N1 will become), we would have no natural immunity to the disease. We could not produce antibodies fast enough to fight the virus (see page 31 for an explanation of this). The number of people suffering complications would be much higher than with seasonal human flu, and it would be likely to affect young, healthy people as well as the elderly and those with existing health problems.

How many people would die of pandemic flu?

This can't be known in advance, but in the UK the minimum number predicted is 53,000 deaths over a three-month period. It could be ten times that number – the mortality rate will depend on lots of factors, including how well people manage to look after themselves and limit the spread of germs. If it is a mild pandemic, it could kill 2 million worldwide. If it is severe, along the lines of the 1918 pandemic, the number could be as high as 150 million.

What are the first symptoms of the lethal strain?

In the cases we have seen in Southeast Asia, the early symptoms have been very similar to common-or-garden flu – a high temperature, coughing and aching muscles. Within three days, however, the patient's breathing has become laboured and they are seriously ill. When the disease becomes fully transmissible between humans, it is likely that it will have its own 'profile' or set of recognizable symptoms – but these may still look like normal flu at first.

TREATMENTS

Can bird flu be treated?

Bird flu can be treated with anti-viral drugs known as neuraminidase inhibitors. The two key drugs at the moment are Tamiflu and Relenza. Both of these can be used preventively, to stop people becoming infected, or they can help to aid recovery once an infection has taken hold. The problem is that there is not currently a large enough supply of the drugs; Britain would quickly use up its whole stockpile if the drugs were prescribed for preventive use. The UK government has ordered 14 million courses of Tamiflu, which would be enough to treat a quarter of the population. However, if a strain of flu develops that is resistant to Tamiflu and Relenza there is currently no other treatment available.

Can anti-viral drugs be given to children?

Yes, anti-viral drugs can be given to children but, as always, need to be prescribed by a doctor to ensure the dose is appropriate for the child's age and size.

How will I get Tamiflu if I am infected?

There are several ways in which you might be able to get access to anti-viral medication. You may need to go to a GP's surgery, or you may receive a home visit from a nurse. Alternatively, drugs may be supplied directly by pharmacists. The government hasn't yet announced what it wants to do.

How quickly do I need to take anti-viral drugs?

These drugs need to be taken fast, within 48 hours of the first symptoms appearing. It isn't documented how well the drugs would work if you took them three or four days after the onset of symptoms.

How can I get a stock of Tamiflu now?

You won't be able to buy the drugs from your local chemist as the manufacturer is keeping back supplies from wholesalers in order to supply different governments around the world. Don't be tempted to buy anti-viral drugs via the Internet. It could be dangerous because you don't know who you're buying from or what the tablets contain. If they're counterfeit, they won't work on the flu virus. You need to consult a health professional before taking Tamiflu, in case it could counteract or have an adverse reaction with any other medication you are taking. Pregnant women should be especially careful to get up-to-date medical advice on the use of medication.

Why don't governments just make more anti-viral medication if it is in such short supply?

There are moves by some countries, such as Thailand, to ask their own pharmaceutical companies to make the anti-viral drugs, but it is quite a complex manufacturing process, and there are all sorts of legal barriers. Roche, which manufactures Tamiflu, has said it will allow other companies to be involved in some parts of the manufacturing process, to speed up the delivery of outstanding orders. Roche say they will have made 300 million courses by the end of 2006, enough to clear the backlog of orders.

Will Tamiflu work for everyone?

No. At best, it may prevent 53 per cent of people from needing hospital care. It does relieve symptoms, but we won't know how well it works until the actual pandemic strain emerges. It's not like an antibiotic, which can completely wipe out a bacterial infection. Tamiflu prevents the virus from spreading throughout the body, but it has to be taken quickly, and it will work better for some people than others. At the moment, there is no way of knowing how

well the anti-viral drugs would work for you if you were infected.

Will I be infectious before I get symptoms?

Yes, probably for one to two days before symptoms begin. Children may be even more infectious and might incubate the disease for several days before you notice the signs.

Will everyone who gets it become seriously ill?

No. The vast majority of people are likely to suffer a very nasty, exhausting bout of flu. They will need to stay at home in bed, drink lots of warm fluids and be looked after by friends or family, but they will not need hospital care. Within a week, they should be over the worst but may feel exhausted for some time after.

Who will get hospital care?

Hospitals will only be able to accept the very sickest patients, because they won't have the staff, the beds or the equipment to care for everyone. Exactly how they will manage the crisis is still being worked out. A shortage of hospital facilities poses the biggest problem for the NHS – but during a pandemic, they could also experience staff shortages when doctors and nurses fall ill.

What if I need other kinds of medical care during a pandemic?

Family doctors and hospitals are attempting to work out how normal services might run during a pandemic. It is likely that routine, non-emergency operations and clinics would be cancelled, but some patients will still need treatment – cancer patients, for example, and those with chronic illnesses like diabetes. These services will have to be safeguarded. There will be an NHS hotline you can ring for help and information.

When will a vaccine be available?

Several possible vaccines are being studied, and some are already in clinical trials. But the problem is that until the virus mutates to become a fully human strain, we don't know exactly what the specific genetic target, or antigen, for the vaccine should be. A vaccine needs to be a very good match for the antigen or it might not work well. The other problem is that there are not enough vaccine factories worldwide to make the quantity of doses we would need.

Once the virus has become a human pathogen, a vaccine can probably be developed within six months, but it may come too late for those hit by the first wave of the pandemic. If we are lucky, a pandemic strain might arrive but not fully take off – so it would give the world time to make a vaccine that could protect enormous numbers of people.

When a vaccine is developed, will it be suitable for children as well as adults?

Yes, the government has made plans for part of the vaccine stockpile to be suitable for children.

Will I be able to get the vaccine from my GP's surgery, and will I have to pay for it?

The first people to get the vaccine will be health workers, police and those running the energy and water supplies. After that, it will go to those thought to be most at risk, which will be those in specific age groups, possibly younger people, and also those with chronic health conditions such as heart problems. The vaccine will be free on the NHS, and immunizations would take place in village halls or town centres, to enable medical staff to vaccinate as many people as possible in a short space of time.

What is the flu vaccine the elderly get every autumn?

This is an immunization against normal, seasonal flu. It will not protect you from bird flu, but it means that if bird flu comes to Britain via our poultry flocks, there will be less chance of the bird flu virus mixing with a human flu strain. It is currently offered to the elderly, those with chronic conditions and those who are susceptible to respiratory infections. It is also offered at some workplaces.

Will those with private healthcare schemes be better placed to get Tamiflu and vaccines?

No. Private medical insurers cannot guarantee their members access to anti-virals or the vaccine.

POULTRY AND PETS

How prevalent is bird flu in British chickens?

Not at all, yet. Extra measures are being taken to monitor the condition of UK poultry and farmers have been given a government helpline number they can phone for advice – or to report anything suspicious.

Can I get bird flu from eating cooked chicken?

No. Both heat and light destroy the virus, and once the meat has been cooked no virus remains. The advice from the Food Standards Agency is to cook chicken thoroughly, just as you would to destroy salmonella bacteria. The UK has stopped importing poultry from affected countries, in any case.

What about eggs?

Eggs are perfectly safe to eat. Again, make sure they are cooked properly. Even if you ate an egg from an infected bird, there would be no risk because your stomach acids would kill off the virus.

Should I be feeding wild birds in my garden and ducks in the park?

The RSPB has said that it is perfectly safe to carry on feeding wild birds, and indeed the birds will need that food to survive over the coming winter months. If you have direct contact with wild birds, it is always wise to wash your hands thoroughly.

Is it still safe to go to nature reserves?

This activity is completely safe in the UK. The wardens on reserves have been told to look out for any unusual deaths among birds so if there was a case of infection, it would be picked up at an early stage. So far, there hasn't been an infected bird in a reserve in Britain.

Are my pets likely to catch bird flu from birds?

It is known that some other animal species can contract the disease, but this won't happen yet as bird flu isn't in the UK. Tests have shown that cats are able to carry the virus, and spread it to other cats. The time to worry about your pets will be when or if bird flu hits Britain, not before. If bird flu does reach the UK, you may wish to consider keeping your pets indoors, especially cats that like to hunt birds.

Are vets well-informed?

All vets have been given information about the disease, and told about the signs to watch out for in birds. Vets will be at the front-line if the disease arrives in birds, so they are very aware of the dangers.

Is it safe to visit a farm at the moment?

Yes, it's as safe as it always was. Farmers are aware of the problems posed by bird flu, and are taking measures to keep their chickens away from any wild birds that might land on their farm. For example, farmers have been told not to feed or water their poultry outdoors any more.

My daughter has a pet budgie. Should I still let her touch it?

As bird flu is not yet present in the UK, it should be fine for children to continue to have contact with their pet birds. Bird flu can infect pet birds, but at present it doesn't pose a threat in the UK. As always, make sure children wash their hands properly after touching pets.

KEEPING POULTRY

Why haven't we banned hen-owners from keeping their birds outdoors, as the French government has?

There's a lot of controversy over whether the government should be more cautious and order all poultry stocks indoors, which is what they have done in some other countries. The Department for the Environment, Food and Rural Affairs (Defra) has adopted a 'wait and see' approach because they say it is too early to adopt such draconian action. But in November 2005 they asked poultry owners to start making preparations which would allow birds to be brought indoors at short notice if an outbreak does occur. Some free-range producers probably couldn't do this because the cost would be too great, and they might have to cull their birds if there was such an order.

Should people who keep chickens in their gardens be worried about bird flu?

No. There is currently no bird flu in Britain. But make sure that you keep your chickens physically separated from any wild birds that may land in the garden. They should have wire over the top of their coop and run so as to prevent them from mixing with wild birds. There is useful advice on the Defra website (see page 216).

I have decided to get rid of our chickens as I'm worried about bird flu. What should I do with them?

Before you do anything, talk to your local vet. If you no longer want them, your vet will advise you how to dispose of them. If chickens have to be culled, it must be done humanely.

Is free-range poultry at a higher risk of bird flu infection than other poultry? If so, is the government going to ban free-range eggs and other free-range products?

Free-range poultry would be at a higher risk if bird flu came to Britain, but the virus isn't here yet. Free-range eggs are extremely popular among consumers and there are currently no plans for a ban.

Will we still be able to get 'free-range' eggs if all hens are locked up?

Under EC rules, it seems that eggs can still be marketed as free-range even if the birds are locked up, but retailers and supermarkets may feel that the descriptions need to be modified. The word 'organic' may no longer apply to eggs or poultry in this situation.

Shouldn't the government be doing more to inform hen owners about the risks?

Defra has sent out guidance to industry bodies, which are trying to inform poultry owners about the risks and how they need to be vigilant for signs of illness in their birds. Apart from messages on their website, they have sent the details to 3,800 veterinary practices around the UK. The problem is that there is no central register for poultry owners, so we don't know how many people keep hens or ducks in their back gardens.

Can we vaccinate birds?

The government could order compulsory vaccination for birds if bird flu arrived in

Britain, but there are problems with this. The main difficulty is that a vaccine would protect birds from dying of the disease, but wouldn't stop them from becoming infected or spreading the virus.

TRAVEL

Is it safe to travel to a country where there have been human cases of bird flu?

Yes, it is perfectly safe to travel to countries where there have been outbreaks of bird flu, but look at page 156 for precautions you might want to take. As the situation develops, the Foreign Office website (see page 216) will give government recommendations about countries that are safe or unsafe to visit.

I'm travelling to Southeast Asia soon and would like to stay with local families in rural regions. Will this put me at risk of bird flu?

This will not put you at risk, as long as you stay at least 1 metre away from any birds and in particular avoid touching them. The greatest danger would be if you were present when a bird was slaughtered, or helped to prepare a meal containing poultry, as this is how many people have caught the infection. Just stay away from birds if you can.

I heard that China will shut its borders if they have a case of human-to-human transmission of bird flu. Should I be worried about travelling there and not being able to leave?

Anyone who travels to a country such as China and then finds themselves subject to this type of restriction would almost certainly be able to come home again if they got in touch with their embassy in that country. There are arrangements for such situations.

If I return from a trip to a country where there have been human cases of the disease and I begin to feel unwell, what should I do?

Go to see your family doctor. Your illness is unlikely to be bird flu, but you should see the doctor in any case, because you might have picked up another infection which needs treatment.

Shouldn't airports be screening people for the disease?

In 2006 we are likely to start seeing more posters going up in airports telling travellers not to get on planes if they feel unwell (see page 135). Staff will also start to look out for people who appear sick. Screening on entry into Britain is pointless until we know that the virus has become a fully human infection.

INTERNATIONAL TRADE

What does 'disease-free status' mean?

This is a term used by the European Union and some other regions to indicate that the disease in question has not been found in that particular country.

Other than protecting the health of their citizens, why are governments so concerned to maintain their country's disease-free status?

Maintaining a disease-free status enables a country to continue exporting its goods to other countries, in the knowledge that they are safe. If a country loses its disease-free status, it is likely that other countries will ban imports of the affected goods (in this case, live poultry and poultry products).

Why has Britain been able to keep its disease-free status when some finches died of bird flu in quarantine?

Because the birds that died were still held in quarantine facilities, they were not officially on UK soil, and therefore we could keep our disease-free status. Luckily, the birds' condition was diagnosed before they were released from quarantine.

Were the birds that died in quarantine from an area already affected by bird flu?

If not, how did they catch the disease?

The finches came from Taiwan, a country that has not reported any cases of bird flu. There is still some confusion over this, with the Taiwanese claiming that the infected birds may have been smuggled in from China. All the birds that were in quarantine with the finches, including the parrot from Surinam that was originally thought to be carrying the disease, have been put down, in order to prevent the virus escaping.

Is our quarantine system good enough to keep out the disease?

The UK's Environment Secretary, Margaret Beckett, has ordered a review of our quarantine procedures specifically to answer this question. A report should be published some time early in 2006.

Will wild birds with the disease eventually bring it to the UK?

There is a possibility this will happen, but it depends how many migratory birds with the virus land on our shores, and then it depends how much opportunity they are given to interact with domestic birds. The UK Department for the Environment, Food and Rural Affairs (Defra) said in November 2005 that the risk had increased recently because of the global spread of the disease, but that it is still low.

Have we banned imports of birds and poultry products from areas that are affected by bird flu?

We have banned imports of live birds and products, such as unprocessed feathers, from counties that have been affected by bird flu, as they could potentially transmit the virus to birds in the UK. A temporary ban on importing captive birds from outside the EU was introduced in October 2005, and this may well become a permanent ban if animal welfare organizations have their way.

What about bird fairs and markets in the UK?

These are under a temporary ban, but there has been no ban on pet shows in general.

What measures will the government take if there is a bird flu outbreak among domestic birds in the UK?

The government has established measures that would be brought into effect quickly if, for example, bird flu was found on a farm. Workers would be given protective suits and vets would go in to cull all birds within a certain radius around the farm. Disinfectant would be widely used on the farm and on vehicles that could carry the virus into other areas.

What measures is the international community taking to slow the spread of bird flu?

Governments around the world are starting to work together to address the bird flu crisis. In Europe, officials have taken part in a simulation exercise to test their readiness for a bird flu pandemic and to see how governments might interact with each other in a crisis. Outside Europe, ASEAN (the Association of Southeast Asian Nations) has launched a three-year plan to address the spread of the virus. And, in November 2005, an international meeting hosted by the WHO, the Food and Agriculture Organization, the World Organization for Animal Health and the World Bank idenitified the key parts of a global action plan to control bird flu and reduce the threat of a human flu pandemic.

SOCIAL MEASURES

Will the government shut schools and other public institutions if bird flu becomes capable of spreading between humans?

When the pandemic is at an early stage, the government may decide to close schools and other public buildings in order to delay the spread of infection within a community. But after a month or so, the disease will be widespread and there may be little point in closing schools. It would damage the economy if parents couldn't get to work because their children were not at school.

What about public transport and shops?

Most retailers intend to stay open, but the key question for them is whether their goods would be able to reach the shops, and that would depend on their suppliers and their drivers, some of whom would be off with flu. Staffing shortages due to illness may mean some retailers are forced to close.

Transport companies will try to keep services running as normally as possible, but trains are likely to be on a reduced service in a pandemic, because many drivers would be off sick. Some companies believe that during a pandemic, nearly half their staff may not make it to work at any one time. See pages 145–148 for ways in which companies are responding to the challenge.

Who will be running the country if there is a bird flu pandemic?

An emergency Cabinet committee will be set up to run services, taking advice from the most senior police officers, health planners and directors of the voluntary services. In each region of Britain, a resilience team has been set up to co-ordinate plans for a pandemic, and they would be expected to oversee local services, such as drug provision, hospitals and the mortuaries. The army could be brought in to help distribute anti-viral drugs and to ensure that food supplies made it through to supermarkets if there were distribution problems.

Will anyone be forced into quarantine if they are infectious?

There has been speculation about this but in practice it's extremely difficult to make people go into quarantine. It would mean the police would have to act as enforcement officers in certain cases, and they will probably be busy with other emergency tasks. People who have been exposed to infection via a family member may be asked to go into voluntary quarantine, particularly at the beginning of the epidemic, to try and slow down the spread of the disease.

STAYING HEALTHY

What are the most important things I can do to protect my health?

There are some simple measures you can take to protect yourself and your family, and these are outlined in Chapter 8. The single most important step you can take is to stop smoking and improve the health of your lungs. Nothing matters more.

Make sure you know how to wash your hands properly and teach your kids the same. It should only take 30 seconds each time. Also teach children to use hankies to cover their nose and mouth when they cough or sneeze. Make sure you eat a healthy diet and get enough sleep and if you are prone to chest infections in winter or you are over 65, go to your GP for a flu jab.

I've seen masks and bird flu emergency kits for sale online. Are these worth buying? Will they help keep me safe if there is a bird flu pandemic amongst humans?

Masks may be useful if you have to use public transport to get to work or attend big meetings, but they must be disposed of carefully in a plastic bag after each journey or meeting. If the masks aren't disposed of carefully, the germs could get get onto your hands. The Health Protection Agency in the UK is not convinced that they would play a major role in protecting people during a pandemic.

Emergency kits might also contain gloves and personal protective suits (PPE). Gloves are a waste of time as handwashing is just as effective, and you won't need a protective suit unless you are a healthcare worker or work on a farm.

GLOSSARY

Adjuvant – a chemical added to a vaccine (see below) that enhances its effects at a lower dosage.

Antibody – a protein made by white blood cells to neutralize antigens (see below) that are introduced to the body.

Antigen – a foreign protein that triggers an immune response in the body, specifically the production of antibodies.

Anti-viral medication – a drug made to combat a virus.

Avian – coming from, or to do with birds.

Bacteria – micro-organisms found in the air, water, foods and the digestive system. Some can cause disease in humans.

Biosecurity – preventive measures taken to stop infection by disease-carrying organisms.

BSE (Bovine Spongiform Encephalopathy) – a nerve disease in cattle that can be passed to humans through infected meat.

CJD (Creutzfeldt-Jakob Disease) – a degenerative disease of the brain, which can be caused by eating meat from cattle suffering from BSE (see above).

Clade – a subsection of a flu genotype (see below) in which the organisms are thought to have developed from a common ancestor.

Clinical attack rate – percentage of the population likely to be infected by a particular virus.

Coronavirus – one of a group of viruses that have a crown-like (corona) shape around them when viewed under a microscope.

DNA (deoxyribonucleic acid) – the main molecule that carries genetic information in most organisms.

Encephalitis – an infection that causes inflammation of the brain, usually caused by a virus.

Enzyme – a protein in the body that regulates chemical reactions, such as digestion.

Epidemiology – a branch of medicine that studies the incidence and distribution of diseases.

Foot-and-mouth disease – a lethal infectious disease in cattle; there was an outbreak in the UK in 2001.

Genotype – the specific genetic make-up of an organism or virus.

GenZ – the dominant genetic form of H5N1.

H1N1 – the flu subtype that caused the 1918–19 pandemic of Spanish flu.

H2N2 – the flu subtype that caused the 1957–8 pandemic of Asian flu.

H3N2 – a human flu virus subtype that can be carried by pigs.

H3N8 – a flu subtype that can be found in horses.

H5N1 – the strain of Asian influenza that is now causing concern.

H7N7 – a subtype that was found in poultry in Holland in 2003.

Haemagglutinin (HA) – one of the key proteins of a flu virus that is able to unlock human cells so the virus can get in to replicate.

Humanized – a term used in association with a virus to mean that it has mutated to become transmissible from human to human, rather than from animal to human.

Immunity – a state when the immune system is able to protect us from disease.

Influenza – an infection of the respiratory tract caused by a virus.

Mortality rate – in the context of diseases, this is the percentage of those who catch a disease that will die because of it.

Mutation – genetic changes in cells as they replicate.

Neuraminidase (NA) – one of the key proteins in a flu virus that is able to unlock human cells so the virus can get in to replicate; it is targeted by the drugs oseltamivir and zanamivir.

Nucleotide – the building blocks of DNA (see above), or RNA (see below).

Orthomyxovirus – one of a family of viruses responsible for respiratory infections, including flu.

Oseltamivir (Tamiflu) – a neuraminidase (see above) inhibitor used as an anti-viral medication to combat flu. Tablets taken orally.

Pandemic – an epidemic that has spread across continents.

Pathogen – a disease-causing organism.

Placebo – a substance given in clinical trials that does not contain any of the active ingredients being tested, so those taking it can be used as a control group.

Pneumonia – a potentially serious inflammation of the lungs, caused by bacteria or viruses.

Polymerase Chain Reaction (PCR) – a method of examining the genetic make-up of an organism.

Prophylaxis – taking drugs or other measures to prevent disease.

Reagent – any chemical substance that takes part in a chemical reaction. Often used to refer to substances used to help analyse what is in a biological sample.

Reassortment – genetic changes that occur when one strain of flu mixes with another and a new strain emerges.

Relenza – see zanamivir.

Reproductive number (RO) – the number of people each infected person is likely to pass the disease on to.

Resistance – in the context of this book it refers to what happens when a disease mutates in such a way that the drugs most commonly prescribed will no longer affect it.

RNA (ribonucleic acid) – a molecule that decodes the genetic information carried by DNA (see above); in some viruses, RNA carries the genetic information.

SARS (severe acute respiratory syndrome) – a serious infection caused by a coronavirus (see above); there was an outbreak in 2003 that was first identified in Hong Kong.

Serotype – the characterization of a micro-organism depending on the antigens (see above) it carries.

'Signature' – the pattern of a particular illness, including the symptoms it typically produces.

Tamiflu – see oseltamivir.

Vaccine – a substance containing a harmless form of a virus or a bacterium, which is given to a person or animal to help them produce immunity (see above) to the disease the organism would cause.

Ventilator – a machine that can help people who are unable to breathe naturally by delivering and expelling air from their lungs.

Virology – the study of viruses.

Virus – a small infectious agent, whose sole purpose is to invade the cells of other organisms and make copies of themselves therein.

Zanamivir – a neuraminidase (see above) inhibitor used as an antiviral medication to combat flu. Breathed in through an inhaler.

Zoonosis – an infectious disease affecting animals, which can in some cases be transmitted to human beings.

USEFUL WEBSITES

INTERNATIONAL

ASEAN (Association of Southeast Asian Nations) Disease Surveillance
www.asean-disease-surveillance.net
Information on the latest bird flu outbreaks and deaths in Asia.

European Health and Consumer Protection Directorate-General
europa.eu.int/comm/food/animal/diseases/controlmeasures/avian/index_en.htm
Information and advice on bird flu, focusing on bird health.

Food and Agriculture Organization of the United Nations (FAO)
www.fao.org/ag/againfo/subjects/en/health/diseases-cards/special_avian.html
Information on bird flu and the international response, with emphasis on its impact on poultry and farming.

World Health Organization
www.who.int
This website includes up-to-date information on outbreaks of avian influenza and the response from the international community. Includes a useful Frequently Asked Questions section.

UK

NHS Direct
www.nhsdirect.nhs.uk
An extremely useful site offering advice and information about all aspects of health.

Department of Environment, Food and Rural Affairs (Defra)
www.defra.gov.uk/animalh/diseases/notifiable/disease/ai/index.htm
Useful information on bird flu for UK residents, including advice
for bird keepers.

Foreign and Commonwealth Office – Avian and Pandemic Flu
www.fco.gov.uk
This website's travel advice section includes a useful fact sheet for
British nationals travelling or living overseas.

Department of Health
www.dh.gov.uk
The Department of Health website offers information on healthcare and different illnesses, including bird flu.

Health Protection Agency
www.hpa.org.uk
Information and advice relating to bird flu, with an emphasis on
its impact on human health and well-being.

The *Lancet*
http://www.thelancet.com/collections/avian_flu
A medical journal with a good collection of articles relating to
bird flu. In depth and thorough.

The *New Scientist*
www.newscientist.com
This is one of the best news organization websites, providing a lot
of science in a digestible form.

Practical Poultry Magazine
www.practicalpoultry.co.uk
Website for a UK-based magazine for poultry enthusiasts. Includes
information on keeping your poultry safe and healthy.

US

Centers for Disease Control and Prevention
www.cdc.gov/flu/avian/index.htm
Information and advice on bird flu.

The National Institute for Allergies and Infectious Diseases
www3.niaid.nih.gov/news/focuson/flu
This institute has been leading much of the research in the US into
bird flu. Good, clear scientific information with diagrams.

AUSTRALIA

Department of Agriculture, Fisheries and Forestry
www.daff.gov.au
Information on the impact of bird flu on farming and industry in
Australia.

Department of Foreign Affairs and Trade – Avian Influenza
Travel Bulletin
www.dfat.gov.au
Advice for Australians visiting countries affected by bird flu.

Department of Health and Ageing
www.health.gov.au/internet/wcms/publishing.nsf/Content/health-
avian_influenza-index.htm
Information and advice for the general public, health professionals, livestock keepers and industry on bird flu.

CANADA

Health Canada
www.hc-sc.gc.ca/iyh-vsv/diseases-maladies/avian-aviare_e.html
Information and advice for Canadian citizens in relation to the bird
flu threat.

Public Health Agency for Canada
www.phac-aspc.gc.ca/influenza/avian_e.html
Information on this site includes reports on wild bird movements
and cases of influenza in ducks, advice for travellers and a useful
question-and-answer section.

NEW ZEALAND

Ministry of Health
www.moh.govt.nz/birdflu
Information on bird flu and New Zealand's national pandemic plan.

New Zealand Food Safety Authority
www.nzfsa.govt.nz/consumers/food-safety-topics/pandemic-influenza/index.htm
Information and advice on pandemic influenza and bird flu.

SOUTH AFRICA

National Institute for Communicable Diseases
www.nicd.ac.za
Information and advice on bird flu.

HONG KONG

Hong Kong Department of Health
www.info.gov.hk/info/flu/eng/index.htm
Information on bird flu and advice on Hong Kong's response.

SINGAPORE

Singapore Government Bird Flu Website
www.birdflu.gov.sg
Features information, answers to questions and the latest news
relating to bird flu.

INDEX

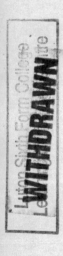